Feet Naturally

By

Dr. Maasi J. Smith

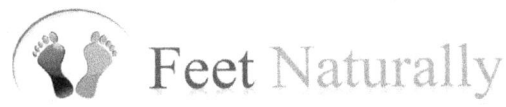

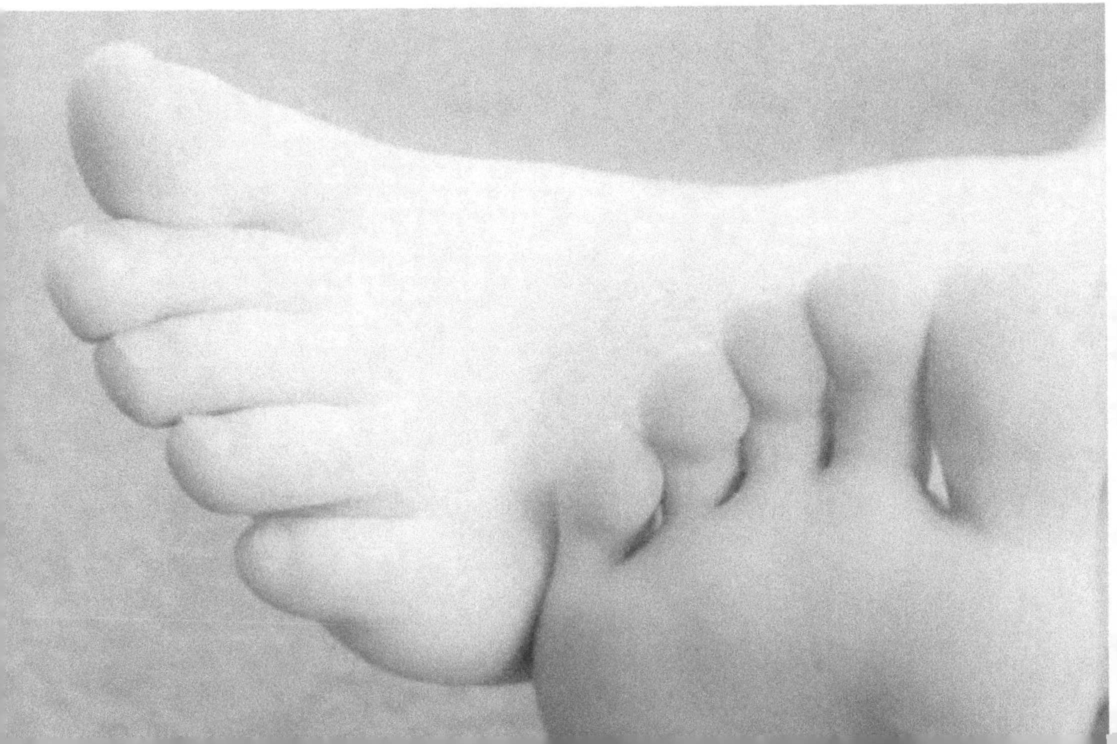

Acknowledgments

Hello, I am Dr. Maasi J Smith, a practicing foot surgeon in Philadelphia, Pennsylvania. I have practiced podiatry* for over a decade. The purpose of *Feet Naturally* is to help people with basic foot problems to find easy, simple natural solutions.

This book is dedicated to all my patients, and staff at Urban Health Initiatives of South Philadelphia.

I would also like to pay tribute to the many friends, organizations and family who have offered their support in all my endeavors. My great mom (Rose M. Smith), and pop (Grady B. Ford) who have always encouraged my best, my Hampton University family, Temple School of Podiatric Medicine's Dean Dr. John Mattiacci, and colleagues, James Wadley PhD, "Good Day" producer Berlinda Garnett, and lastly my very best friend Dominique Casimir Smith.

A special dedication to my wonderful daughters Noelle and Nyla.

Thank you to my editors Grace Campbell, Liji Thomas MD, and Keri Wehlander.

Photography: Cover & Back – Whitney Thomas

STOP AND READ!

Table of Contents

Chapter 1

Introduction

Our feet are often the most neglected part of our body. Incidentally, they are also the part most exposed to daily trauma. An average individual takes 7,000-10,000 steps each day. Thus, the feet naturally tend to collect germs and dirt. They take a beating every day of our lives starting the day we learn to walk.

When you think about your foot, you need to treat it well as an important part of your anatomy. The human foot and ankle is a strong, complex structure containing 26 bones, 33 joints, and more than a hundred muscles, tendons*, and ligaments*. It is important to take daily care of your feet. An unkempt and untended foot can harbor many fungal and bacterial diseases. Neglect can also result in structural issues like bunions, hammer toes, and heel pain. So treat your feet well in order to protect them.

How frequently do you wash your feet after a day of work or exercise? You should spend at least fifteen minutes soaking your feet in a tub of warm, soapy water. This simple step will not only keep your feet clean but also rejuvenate them by de-stressing tensed muscles.

Every season, the human body goes through physical changes. Feet are exposed to the effects of the weather, and therefore experience physical changes, such as tanning, cracks and fissures. In the summer months, we generally take to wearing open footwear like flip-flops*, sandals*, floaters*, and slippers*, so it is vital to keep your feet in good condition during this season.

Alternate your shoes each day. Feet sweat, so it's important to let shoes dry out completely

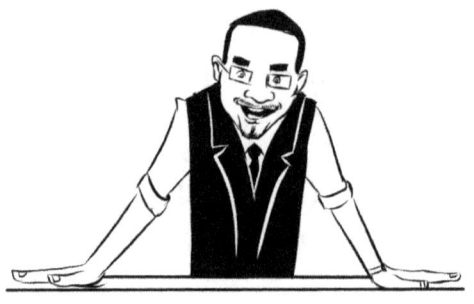

Summer is a sweaty and humid season in most areas. Even in areas with low humidity and hot weather, your feet will still sweat. You can prevent the accumulation of sweat by dusting your feet freely with an anti-fungal foot powder. The powder acts as an excellent sweat absorber. This keeps your feet dry and also keeps foot pores from being blocked, thus allowing your feet to breathe. This is vital in preventing fungal infection.

To avoid tanning issues like darkening and discoloration, use a good quality sunscreen* to protect them from the harmful UV* rays of the sun. If you have sweaty or oily skin, choose a water-based tanning lotion that is compatible with your skin texture. If you wear closed footwear such as sneakers and shoes, remember to dust the insides with powder so the shoes don't smell or accumulate sweat.

Winters might be expected to be less damaging, as the feet are usually kept covered. But covering them is not enough; your feet need frequent moisturizing*, as the skin tends to dry out. This keeps cracks and fissures from developing. Massage them with a good moisturizing cream to keep the skin hydrated and supple. Don't ignore cracked heels and soles. If you expose them to cold dry air and neglect early signs of skin drying and cracking, serious foot infections could result. It is always better to treat these symptoms at once, while they are still in the early stages. Rehydrate your feet by using moisturizer* regularly and wear soft cotton or woolen socks afterwards, as the extra protection will help to accelerate healing.

Many men think of grooming as a sissy trait. The truth is that cleanliness is important for both men and women. Men need to remember that good grooming includes a healthful approach to body hygiene and care.

Basic body hygiene needs to be part of everyone's routine on a daily basis. This doesn't mean that you have to visit expensive spas* or luxurious salons* every day. There are many natural and homemade ingredients around you that have amazing properties to help you care for yourself, and especially for your feet. By bringing more attention to your feet, you will actually benefit all of your wonderful body.

Once in a while, it's fun to treat yourself to a pedicure* or a professional foot treatment to provide extra care for your feet. But it is also important that you set up a daily foot care routine to keep your feet in good condition. In the following chapters, I will discuss problems related to feet in general, as well as their causes and the various natural remedies available for these conditions. I have also provided some information related to feet conditions so my readers may be more aware of the importance of foot care.

Some Interesting Facts about the Human Foot:

- Each human foot contains twenty-six bones and has more than a hundred ligaments.
- Both feet together make up more than a fourth of the number of bones in the human body.
- The skin of the feet contains more than seven thousand nerve endings.
- There are over 250,000 sweat glands in the skin of each foot, which together produce half a cup of sweat every day.

Chapter 2

Natural Home Remedies For Common Foot Problems

This chapter deals with some common foot problems and available natural remedies to treat them. I have chosen to deal with the kind of foot problems that most of us face at some point in our lives, mostly due to neglect and lack of foot care. These problems should never be ignored and allowed to become serious. For this reason, I have indicated which natural remedial measures will help overcome these run-of-the-mill foot problems.

PROBLEM 1:	ACHILLES TENDONITIS

The Achilles tendon is the largest tendon in the human body, as well as the one most commonly ruptured. It is found behind the ankle joint and connects the calf muscles to the heel. Achilles tendonitis* is a condition in which this structure overstretches due to sudden or excessive strain. The tendon typically becomes painful at its insertion, at the back of the heel. The most common causes of this condition include sports injuries and other strenuous physical activities, such as:

- Intense exercise like running, jogging, or power walking that puts excessive strain on the calf muscles.
- Not warming up properly before a vigorous exercise session, which can put a lot of strain on your calf muscles and cause the tendon to tear.
- Climbing staircases or steep hills can cause the Achilles tendon to become sore.
- A sudden pull or trauma to the calf muscles can result in the irritation of this tendon.
- Ill-fitting footwear and flat feet can also lead to Achilles tendonitis.

Symptoms of Achilles Tendonitis

- A subtle pain in the calf area that gradually worsens with continued exertion of the calf muscles.
- Severe pain in the calf region, limited to the region of the upper back portion of the heel, and appearing on continuous exertion.
- Pain, swelling, and tenderness occurring especially in the morning in the area just below the calf muscles (at the back, where the Achilles tendon joins the heel bone).
- A feeling of heaviness in the affected area, causing slowness while walking.
- Stiffness, which gradually disappears as you warm up or become active.

Treatment for Achilles Tendonitis

The best treatment for Achilles tendonitis is usually giving the feet ample time to rest. You can reduce the symptoms markedly just by wrapping a firm bandage around the painful area, to restrict the movement of the tendon. There are also some herbal remedies that can provide significant relief.

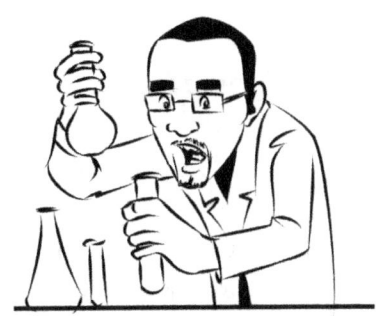

Hydrate the skin using lotions and creams regularly.

Warm oil massage - Massage your calves down to the heel with essential oils* like eucalyptus, peppermint, cardamom, and camphor. These essential oils speed up the healing of your tendon. Avoid all forms of heavy exercise, but keep your legs flexible by doing light activities like swimming or stretching, which are not likely to harm or stress the tendon.

Achilles tendonitis generally heals at home with these natural treatments, along with rest, ice and elevation. But if you have severe pain or other symptoms, it is advisable to get a medical evaluation. In more serious cases, a rupture or tear may be present that may require surgical repair.

PROBLEM 2:	ANKLE SPRAIN

An ankle sprain is when the ligaments holding the ankle bones together are stretched excessively during a twisting motion at the ankle. The ligaments on the outside of the ankle are most commonly affected. Sprains may be mild or severe depending on the intensity and number of ligaments involved.

Symptoms

Ankle sprains are characterized by acute pain in the ankle area, followed by redness, soreness, swelling, and bruising. If the sprain is severe, there may be significant pain and dark bruising around the foot and ankle area.

Treatment

An easy way to remember what you should do for such injuries is the acronym RICE, which stands for: Rest, Ice, Compression (bandage), and Elevate. Because of the prolonged period of rest that an ankle sprain requires, the muscles around the ankle often become shortened and tight. Ankle rehabilitation after a sprain needs to be done carefully.

Ice Packs and Elevation

An ankle sprain produces inflammation of the area. Ligaments are stretched and bruised and the blood rushes to the area to help it heal. If an ankle is sprained, avoid putting any weight on it. Elevate it to encourage the swelling to go down.

Putting an ice pack on it immediately helps diminish injury. The ice slows down the blood flow to the injury and will keep the swelling down. But wrap the ice pack in a towel and move it around: it should not stay in one place. And alternate twenty minutes on with twenty minutes off. When icing the injury, keep it elevated above heart level.

A very gentle massage of the sprained area with essential oils like peppermint and camphor provides great relief. These oils have a cooling and calming effect on your sore ankle and help reduce swelling and inflammation*.

The next step is to wrap a support bandage around the injured ankle. This will support it and speed up the rate of healing. A serious ankle sprain may need surgical intervention to repair torn and/or damaged ligaments. Such serious sprains are usually seen in sports injuries.

Soak in Epsom Salt*

Epsom salts are made up of minerals such as magnesium. When dissolved in warm water, these are absorbed into the skin and replenish lost minerals in your body. It will also ease the pain and relieve inflammation. Add a cupful of the salt to a basin of warm water and soak until the water cools. You can also make a compress by wrapping the sprain with a cloth that has been soaked in Epsom salt solution.

Drink Tea

If you are healing well, and don't require prescription medications, try herbal teas, such as green tea or chamomile, which are fantastic for reducing inflammation.

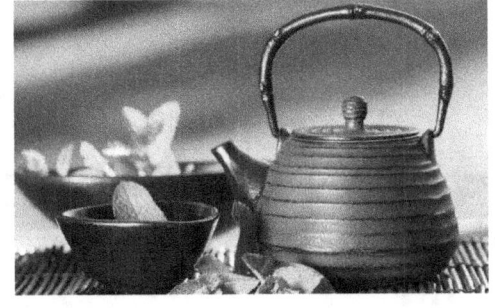

If you sprain your ankle repeatedly, you need to change your footwear. Store bought ankle supports and straps will help. Padded shoes with arch supports are also useful, but make sure they give your feet good support and balance. Exercise your feet and ankles to keep them strong, as well as to speed up healing. Start with non-weight bearing exercises (bike riding, swimming), then move to resistance exercises. A physical therapist will guide you through these.

PROBLEM 3:   ARTHRITIS

Arthritis is the medical term for joint inflammation. There are more than a hundred variants of this condition, most of which have no cure. However, you can learn to manage them with proper preventive and care measures. Arthritis can also occur when bone has lost cartilage due to disease or overuse. Cartilage covers the bone surface to stop the two bones from rubbing directly against each other. The covering of cartilage allows the joint to work smoothly and painlessly. If this cartilage is lost, bone on bone contact occurs, causing significant pain. In these cases natural treatments can only help with the symptoms; your physician will advise you on definitive treatment.

Symptoms

The disease usually manifests with tenderness, swelling and redness, inflammation, stiffness, pain in the joints, and restricted movement in the affected areas. Arthritis readily responds to natural home remedies.

Natural Home Remedies for Arthritis

Arthritis is an incurable illness and can cause unbearable pain at times. However, the following natural home remedies can provide a great measure of relief. If you consistently take preventive steps and apply natural remedies as and when called for, you can deal with your condition very effectively.

Hot Compression - If you have hot, red and swollen joints, or acute arthritis, you should avoid heat application. Otherwise, hot packs are one of the most valuable pain relief techniques for people suffering from arthritis. Soothing hot compresses can work wonders on painful joints and muscles, relieving pain, reducing muscle stiffness, and improving the circulation. You can use soft, thick towels soaked in hot water, hot water bags, heating pads*, or electric blankets to apply heat. You may also consider rubbing the painful joints with essential oils, like eucalyptus and camphor oils, which generate warmth and ease the pain.

Buy proper size shoes. Shop late in the day when feet tend to be at their largest.

Cold Compression - Cold compresses are the best way to relieve arthritic joints that are severely inflamed or feel hot, sore, and painful. Applying cold compresses to the affected area markedly relieves pain and inflammation of the joints and muscles, such as in acute gout or Raynaud's phenomenon*. Cold compresses can be applied in the form of a towel soaked in ice-cold water or running water, an ice pack, or a bag of frozen peas. However, you should be careful to wrap frozen bags or ice packs in a towel before application to avoid frostbite to the area.

Alternate Soaks – The best and most effective way to relieve arthritis is the technique of alternating hot and cold soaks. This stimulates circulation, reduces pain and swelling, and de-stiffens joints. This method has been recommended by the Arthritis Foundation. Their guidelines specify that the hot water should not be at a temperature more than 110 ° F, while the temperature of the cold water should be around 65 ° F. The warm soak may last about 3 minutes, while the cold soak should last only a minute.

Shoe Size – Buying shoes of the proper size is very important. Shoes can contribute to pain and discomfort by being too tight or too loose. You may have two feet that are slightly different in size and shape, and your feet can actually have different measurements at different times of the day.

Another thing to avoid is assuming your feet are still the same size as your old shoe. Most feet gradually widen with age, and sometimes women's feet "grow" after having a child due to muscle relaxation during pregnancy.

Shop for shoes in the late afternoon or evening, since that's when your feet are the biggest. Feet tend to swell during the day. Have the salesperson measure both feet while you're standing up as your feet will expand under the weight of your body. You want 1/3 to 1/2 an inch in front of your big toe to allow your feet to spread. This toe space is important because proper shoe size can significantly reduce the pain of arthritis, bunions and hammer toes as well as general foot pain.

Epsom Salts - Epsom salts (magnesium sulfate salt) work well to relieve general pain and inflammation. Mix a generous quantity of Epsom salts in a tub of warm water (1 tablespoon per ½ gallon of water) and soak your aching arthritic feet in it for a while. Use it in your bath as well to ease general bodily aches and pains.

Eucalyptus Oil* - This pungent essential oil is a potent pain reliever. It has natural warming properties. For the best results, massage the affected area daily with warmed eucalyptus oil, followed by hot compresses, preferably before bedtime. A mixture of eucalyptus and wintergreen oil can be used as well.

Borage Seed Oil* - Borage seed oil is another great option for treating arthritic pain. Borage seed oil has potent anti-inflammatory properties that can reduce pain and swelling in the inflamed joints. When it is massaged into the painful area regularly, it can help reduce joint swelling. This oil can also be used internally (one teaspoon a day) to help relieve arthritis pain.

Turmeric* – Turmeric is a very common kitchen spice, but has remarkably valuable antiseptic and anti-inflammatory properties. It is very useful in treating arthritic inflammation and pain. About 1500 mg to 3000 mg of turmeric should be consumed daily to relieve the symptoms of arthritis. This can be in the form of a cup of fresh turmeric juice to start off your day. A tablespoon of turmeric powder in a glass of warm water or milk is also a good bedtime drink that helps reduce arthritic pain.

Ginger - Ginger is another kitchen ingredient that is a very good treatment for arthritis. The anti-inflammatory properties of ginger help reduce the pain, swelling, tenderness, and stiffness of arthritis drastically. Ginger also aids in improving the circulation of blood in the body. Ginger oil is useful for massaging into the painful area. Or include raw ginger in your diet to stimulate internal healing. Boil some fresh grated ginger in water and use the water to soak your feet once it has cooled to a comfortable temperature. If you are diabetic you may suffer from numbness in your feet (neuropathy*), and so you should always take precautions to avoid burns from the hot water. Test the water temperature with your elbow or the back of your hand. Even better, ask your podiatrist before soaking your feet.

Cinnamon - Cinnamon is also a good pain reliever. You may massage the painful area with cinnamon oil every day, or you can make a refreshing anti-inflammatory drink from a teaspoon of cinnamon powder mixed with honey and warm water to be taken on an empty stomach every morning.

Some Useful Tips for Managing Arthritis

- Maintaining joint movement is an essential part of dealing with arthritis. Keep your joints flexible by working out daily. Exercise also helps reduce the risk of injury to the joints, but you should be careful not to go overboard. Too strenuous a workout can cause serious secondary damage to arthritic joints. Light workouts such as walking, swimming or easy gardening are best to keep your joints supple. There are also many special exercises for arthritic patients that can keep your joints supple if performed regularly.

Another tip is to maintain an ideal body weight. Being overweight puts great pressure on your heels and foot joints. Weight reduction will provide drastic pain relief, take much of the strain off your feet, and improve your overall health.

Avoid taking part in strenuous activities that put pressure on your joints. Instead, take up activities that spread the strain over a larger area so that arthritic joints are less stressed. For example, cycling and swimming are low impact, but still very effective in providing full body workouts.

Change your posture at regular and brief intervals to prevent excessive bony/muscular strain and stiffening of the joints. Whether you are sitting or standing, stretch your limbs from time to time to relieve joint pain and stimulate circulation. When you climb stairs, always make sure your stronger leg leads, but when you are coming down, lead with your weaker leg. This will not only prevent falls but will ensure your joints are not overstressed.

PROBLEM 4:   **ATHLETE'S FOOT**

Athlete's foot is a very common condition. It is simply a fungal infection of the skin over the feet and usually affects the skin between the toes, slowly spreading to other areas. You will usually experience a burning sensation in the area, with intense itching, small red blisters, inflammation and scaly, cracked skin. It can also be asymptomatic, when it looks like just persistent dry skin.

Since athlete's foot is a contagious disease, the spores* can easily spread from objects used by a person who has it. The disease can be transmitted to other parts of the body as well, since it has a tendency to spread. If the infection is allowed to become very severe, the foot becomes painful and swollen.

What Causes Athlete's Foot?

The organism responsible for athlete's foot is a fungus called tinea pedis. Since fungi thrive in moist places, these breed in public showers or bathrooms. Athlete's foot occurs when tinea pedis grows on the skin of your feet. The same fungus may also grow on the heels, palms, and between the fingers. It can quickly transfer to the skin by walking barefoot in an infected area or using an infected towel. Closed shoes can harbor this infection due to the hot, humid conditions. Walking barefoot can expose your feet to much more than tinea pedis and is a dangerous thing to do.

Natural Remedies for Athlete's Foot

If the condition is mild, athlete's foot can be treated with any of a number of home remedies. However, if you have severe symptoms of athlete's foot (cracking, itching and burning), you should seek medical help. The following are some natural remedies for mild athlete's foot.

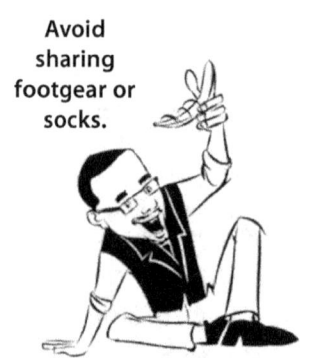

Avoid sharing footgear or socks.

You can get fungal infections by wearing other peoples' footwear.

Tea Tree Oil – This oil, extracted from the leaves of Melaleuca alternifolia, is a highly effective antifungal agent. Just apply the oil to the affected part several times a day for a week or two for amazing results. The oil kills the fungal growth from the base up, resulting in complete healing. If you use this oil regularly, you will never have to fear this infection. One of the strongest antifungals available, its efficacy exceeds even that of prescription drugs. It is best used undiluted, but can be an irritant to the skin. There are diluted versions available which might be safer options.

Garlic – This humble spice doubles as a potent antifungal, and is active against a variety of fungal infections. Many ancient antifungal and antibacterial preparations include garlic as an ingredient. You just need to rub a clove of it on the infected area, or alternatively, mix a crushed garlic clove with a few drops of tea tree oil and rub it gently on the affected area. Once the paste dries, wash it off and then dust it dry with antifungal powder.

Thyme - This herb is very useful in treating fungal and bacterial infections. It is a good antiseptic with antifungal properties as well. It can be applied in the fresh form, in dried powder, or as essential oil, with equally good effects.

Apple Cider Vinegar - Mix one part of apple cider vinegar, four parts of warm water, and half a cup of Epsom salts in a tub and soak your feet in it. Apple cider vinegar helps to create an acidic environment that prevents the growth of fungal infections.

Cinnamon - Boil a generous quantity of cinnamon bark in water until the flavor starts emanating from the steam. Allow the water to sit until it cools to a comfortable warmth. Soak your feet in the warm water. Cinnamon has amazing antiseptic properties that prevent the fungus from re-infecting your feet. Use daily or according to your need.

Yogurt – This is one of the most effective antibacterial foods. It contains live acidophilus bacteria that actively fight yeast/fungal infections of any kind. Apply a generous quantity of yogurt daily on the affected area for amazing results. It also soothes the irritating symptoms of itching and burning, giving you considerable relief.

Tea - Tea is another excellent ingredient in fighting athlete's foot. It contains tannic acid, which alleviates the burning and itching associated with athlete's foot and destroys the fungus as well. Put 8 to 10 bags of black tea in a tub of warm water, put your feet in, and let them soak until the water cools.

Salt – Add a few tablespoons of salt to a tub of warm water and soak your feet for about 15 minutes. Dab your feet dry with a towel and then dust some baking soda on your feet to help absorb excess moisture. Remember, fungi thrive in moist environments.

PROBLEM 5:   BLISTERS

Blisters are small bumps filled with water that develop when your skin keeps rubbing against something. When you wear ill-fitting shoes, your feet will show signs of blister formation. The skin first becomes red and tender, then sore, and finally, blisters pop up. The excessive friction caused by tight footwear which injures the skin.

Blister Symptoms

- Pain and warmth in the affected area
- Burning sensation
- Thin-walled, tender swelling filled with watery fluid
- Redness and irritation

Natural Home Remedies for Treating Blisters

Since blisters are due to abnormal friction on the skin, the first thing to do is to reduce whatever behavior is causing the blisters to form. There are a number of excellent natural remedies for this condition, some of which I have listed below.

Soak the affected blister in warm water once a day for 15 minutes. This will help to clean out the blister, allowing it to drain and eventually dry up.

You can apply antibiotic ointment to a foot blister to promote healing and prevent infection. You also can mix a teaspoon of antibiotic ointment to one gallon of warm water and soak the affected area for 15 to 20 minutes. A one-time soak should be sufficient to heal the blister.

Homemade Blister Foot Powder - In a blender, combine a half-cup of white talcum powder, a half-cup of cornstarch powder, a quarter-cup of powdered peppermint leaves, a quarter-cup of powdered sage leaves, and a half-teaspoon of clove essential oil. Once blended, the mix can be stored in a cool, dry place. Dust the powder on your blistered feet and in your socks as well. It has high absorbency and will soak up moisture and keep friction at bay by lubricating the skin.

Homemade Blister Foot Cream – In a bowl, whisk together a half-cup of vegetable shortening, a teaspoon of eucalyptus oil, and a teaspoon of peppermint or camphor oil. Store the blended mixture in a small glass or plastic container and refrigerate. Use it on the affected areas every day. Remember to wear thick socks after application to reduce friction between your shoes and your feet.

PROBLEM 6:   BUNIONS

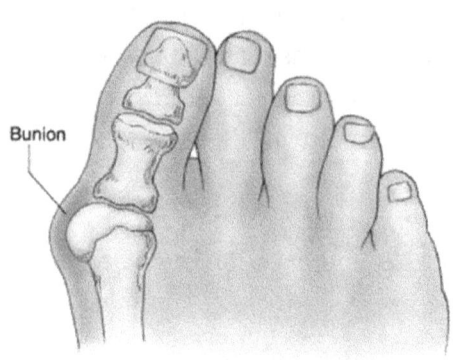

Bunion

Bunions are red, painful, bony bumps that appear generally on the inner side of the base of the big toes. They chiefly occur due to the extended use of tight shoes that constrict the toes, or due to faulty foot structures (genetics). Bunions can cause great pain and discomfort, making surgical correction a necessity.

Symptoms of Bunions

Bunions are typically painful and induce symptoms like reddening, burning, stinging pain, discomfort, aching, and inflammation. It is also possible to have bunions of any size and have no pain.

Natural Home Remedies for Treating Bunions

Treating bunions at home is difficult because bunions are structural deformities, and therefore typically need surgical care. The following home treatments can provide some relief to bunion pain. However, if your symptoms linger even after you have tried natural remedies, it would be best to seek medical advice from your podiatrist.

Application of Cold Compression or Ice Pack - Use cold compresses or an ice pack several times a day for at least ten minutes at a time on your bunions. This usually provides great relief and comfort.

Aloe Vera* Gel – You could try applying aloe vera gel on the affected area to soothe the burning and irritation. Aloe vera is a potent antiseptic with superb anti-inflammatory properties. If you happen to have an aloe vera plant at home, cut a piece off the fleshy leaf and rub the exposed gel-like interior on the bunion.

Some Additional Tips to Deal with Bunions

1. Wear floaters or flip-flops since they have a good arch support system. This helps reduce the pressure on your toes. Make sure the flip-flops you buy are comfortable and well-fitting, and have good supporting straps to support your toes. Be sure to wear them all the time so your big toes are always protected.
2. Use a gel or silicone toe spreader* while wearing your flip-flops. The spreader provides a soft padded support to the toe that has the bunion. Some flip-flops even come with inbuilt gel-padded systems positioned strategically inside the straps to help reduce friction while walking.
3. Selecting a good pair of socks is also important when you have bunions. Socks act to reduce friction and provide a cushioned support to your painful bunions. There are many custom-made socks available that are designed for this condition, and they will act much better than your regular ones to give your bunions maximum protection.
4. Use special bunion pads* made from silicone or gel to give padded protection to your big toes.

5. There are also toe separators* and splints available for bunions, which you can place between your toes to protect them from rubbing against each other. These toe separators are available in both gel* and silicone* forms.
6. Use special stretchable shoes for bunions. These unique shoes are designed to be elastic to provide great comfort and breathing space for your feet. They also help greatly reduce the pressure on your toes.

PROBLEM 7:   BURNING FEET

Burning feet can be caused by neuropathy, or nerve damage. Damaged nerve fibers can become overactive and misfire on their own. This causes pain signals to the brain, although there is no wound or injury.

In most people with neuropathy, the foot nerves tend to become damaged first, because they are the at the farthest part of the body and are also subject to constant and repeated stress during walking, running and so on.

Diabetes is the most common cause of neuropathy and burning feet. However, other conditions also can cause this condition including but not limited to: chronic kidney disease, alcohol abuse, Lyme disease, HIV/AIDS, edema, fluid retention due to hypertension, and vitamin B deficiency.

You may be sensitive to the fabric, leather or dye in your shoes or socks, or the detergent used to wash your socks. Try different kinds of socks, made of different materials. Change your detergent for mild organic soap.

Natural Treatment

Burning feet can be soothed effectively in your home. Essential oils like peppermint oil, eucalyptus oil, camphor oil, lavender oil, and almond oil use counterirritant stimulation to soothe burning feet. Almond oil is especially beneficial in cases where the burning sensation is due to vitamin B deficiency. Massage it into the skin daily for 5-10 minutes.

PROBLEM 8:   CALLUSES

Calluses are hard thickened areas on the feet that result from the accumulation of layers of dead skin on the foot. Sometimes they can become quite large. Calluses occur when continuous and prolonged pressure is applied to a particular part of the foot. This eventually cuts off the circulation, and so the skin layers die. As the dead skin piles up, a callus forms. The most common sites are the heels, which bear most of the weight of the body. Some calluses are deeply seated due to excessive pressure. They may cause pain and discomfort and even restrict your mobility. The primary causes for callus formation are obesity, high-heeled shoes, flat feet, high arched feet, excessive foot pressure and deformed feet.

Natural Remedies and Prevention

There are many natural remedies and preventions for treating calluses. But the most important step is to first eliminate the root cause of the formation of calluses.

Appropriate Body Weight - Maintain an ideal body weight so your feet do not have to bear excessive pressure and strain.

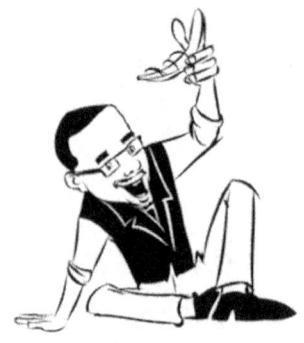

Avoid walking barefoot.

Avoid Improper Shoes – Women especially need to use the right footwear. Avoid using uneven shoes, high heels, or sloping platform shoes. Wearing this kind of footwear for a long time can seriously and permanently damage the structure of your feet. You might require surgery later on for correction.

Padded Footwear - Use padded or orthotic* footwear, which helps distribute foot pressure evenly over your feet, providing safe support. You will find that once the pressure on the calluses is taken off, they will slowly heal by themselves.

Moisturize your Feet – Apply moisturizer generously and give your feet a long warm water soak, so that the calluses are gradually peeled off layer by layer. If you have patience and the will to take care of your feet, you can scrub off your calluses bit by bit in the privacy of your home.

You should never ever try to cut off the dead skin with a blade or other sharp instrument, as it could lead to cuts and ulcers. A cut in the skin could introduce an infection, either bacterial or fungal, and lead to a non-healing wound. Diabetics beware!

Do you like going to the beach? Walking on wet sand can work well on this condition. Wet sand acts as an abrasive* that will help remove the layers of dead skin that make up corns and calluses.

Callus Treatment Using Baking Soda - Add 1 tablespoon of baking soda to a foot spa, basin, or anything your feet can soak in. Fill it halfway with warm water and soak your feet for at least half an hour. Then, with a pumice* stone, carefully file away the hardened skin.

Treating Foot Calluses with Aspirin - Grind six aspirin tablets into a powder. Add half a teaspoon of lemon juice and half a teaspoon of water. Stir the mixture together until you have a thick paste. Apply the paste to the calluses and wrap your foot in a warm towel. Then place it inside a plastic bag. The combination of the warmth and the paste will begin to break down the calluses. Leave your foot inside the bag for 15 minutes. Remove the bag and towel. The calluses will be extremely soft. Now you can file them down successfully with an emery* board or pumice stone.

Epsom Salt - Another good way to soften calluses is to soak them in a foot spa* of water containing a few tablespoons of Epsom salt. Soak for 10-15 minutes to help soften calluses and also deal with foot odor.

Vinegar - Cotton balls soaked in vinegar may be taped to the callus. Allow them to stay on overnight. In the morning, the area will be soft. Scrub with a pumice stone. Be careful not to be overly aggressive when using the pumice stone, as you may scrape and damage your skin.

Cornstarch - Moisture will make the calluses feel more uncomfortable and promote fungal infections. To help reduce some of the discomfort from calluses, sprinkle cornstarch on your feet liberally. This will keep them dry and protect the skin from breaking down. It will also reduce foot odor as a bonus.

PROBLEM 9:   CAPSULITIS

Capsulitis is inflammation of a joint capsule. Ligaments sur-
round your bodily joints, including your toe joints, and help
form a capsule. Joint capsules help your joints to function properly. Capsulitis can also cause inflammation of the ligament that
joins the toe bones to the metatarsal* bone. Causing pain in the
'balls of the feet". It usually results from injury or undue pressure, which may occur in steep climbing, wearing high-heeled
shoes, and performing toe-bending activities like dancing, running and aerobics.

Symptoms

The symptoms often include mild or severe pain in the front
foot as well as discomfort and uneasiness during movement.

Remedy

This condition usually clears up with
rest. You could also try a gentle massage with eucalyptus or peppermint oil
to reduce the pain. Avoid high heels or
ill-fitting shoes, as these put unnecessary strain on your feet. Instead, opt to
wear flat level shoes that have strong
heel support. If you have severe symptoms, you should seek medical help.

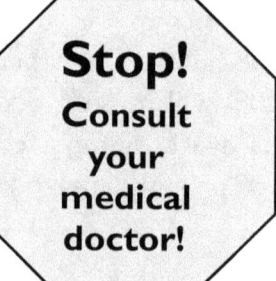

Stop!
**Consult
your
medical
doctor!**

PROBLEM 10:   COLD FEET

Cold feet result from the poor circulation of blood in the body. It is common in those who are anemic or have weakened immunity.

While cold feet are usually not serious medical problems, they can be troublesome. They cause not only discomfort but painful chilblains* and prickly bumps on the skin. Exposure to cold and heightened cold sensitivity can give rise to similar symptoms in peripheral parts of the body like the nose, fingers, and ears.

This condition can be treated naturally at home and does not require any medication unless accompanied by other serious health complications. There are many natural home remedies for treating cold feet, which, when carefully applied, can prove to be of immense benefit in relieving the discomfort.

Some Common Causes of Cold Feet

- Cold feet can be caused by undue exposure to cold temperatures. Sudden temperature changes can also trigger this condition.
- It can also be caused by the poor circulation of blood in the body or anemia.
- Serious health conditions like cardiovascular disease, hypothyroidism*, diabetic neuropathy, multiple sclerosis*, hormonal changes, and genetic conditions may also cause cold feet.
- Raynaud's syndrome is another physical condition that can cause cold feet. This condition is characterized by

vasospastic attacks, or periods of constriction of the blood vessels, which mainly affect the feet and hands. The resulting numbness, paleness, and coldness of the fingers and toes is uncomfortable or even painful. Women are more affected than men. Emotional stress, exposure to cold, or smoking can cause the condition to worsen. Some anti-migraine or anti-hypertensive medications can trigger cold feet, because they act to constrict the blood vessels and so reduce circulation.

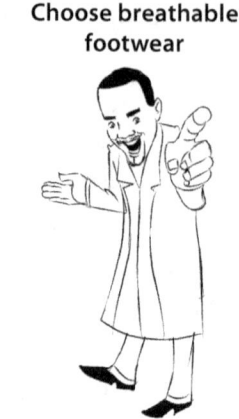

Choose breathable footwear

- Cold feet can also happen without any obvious physical problem.

Symptoms of Cold Feet

- The affected person has a disturbing and uncomfortable sensation of coldness in the hands and feet, which also look pale and feel numb. During an attack, your feet may turn bluish-green or become pale white.

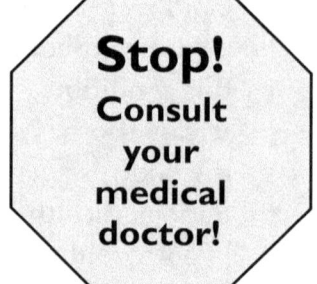

Stop! Consult your medical doctor!

- Other symptoms that may accompany cold feet are swelling, itching, burning, and pain in the feet.
- Blisters may also occur, and may cause itching and discomfort.

Natural Home Remedies for Cold Feet

Massage - Massaging is one of the most effective natural remedies for cold feet. This is because massaging stimulates the blood vessels and capillaries, and so increases the blood flow to your feet as well as creating warmth. Rubbing your feet with eucalyptus oil, ginger oil, jojoba oil, or wheat germ oil is even better. Eucalyptus in particular is known to provide almost instant heat, warming up the cold skin. A mixture of ginger, jojoba, and wheat germ oil also works great in this condition. After a thorough massage with one of these, let your feet soak for some time in warm water and then pat dry.

Therapeutic Oil Mix – Another effective essential oil mixture is a combination of warm almond oil, rosemary oil, and black pepper oil. This should be worked well into the foot's skin by massaging. It produces a sensation of warmth in cases of cold feet.

Hot Footbath – Another simple but effective remedy for cold feet is to soak your feet in a tub of warm water after adding a few drops of peppermint oil, tea tree oil, ginger oil, cypress oil, or any essential oil you like. There's nothing like a warm foot bath to soothe your skin, warm up your feet, and calm your spirit.

Epsom Salt – This very common and popular ingredient of beauty products is also excellent for cold feet. Mix some Epsom salt in a tub of warm water and let your feet soak in the warmth. However, be sure not to use very hot water, which strips your skin of its own natural oils, and may give you chilblains.

Foot Exercise – Foot exercises are the last word in improving foot circulation. This leads to warm feet – naturally. A couple of effective exercises for cold feet are:

Bouncing on your toes and heels for some time is a great way to relieve cold feet.

Activities like walking, cycling, hiking, running, and dancing are also useful in this condition.

Foot Pack – If you have cold feet, try your own foot pack. Combine 2 cups of warm water, one teaspoon of olive oil, a half teaspoon of orange essential oil, a half cup of honey, a cup of freshly minced ginger, powdered oats, cinnamon powder, and cayenne pepper powder. Mix the ingredients into a thick paste and apply liberally on both feet. After half an hour, wash off with lukewarm water. Your feet will feel warm and comfortable.

Cayenne* Pepper - This is an ingredient that greatly stimulates blood flow to your feet. Dust a little cayenne pepper powder into your socks before you wear them to experience instant foot warming. The inherent heat of this spice increases blood circulation. Prolonged use of this can stain your socks and shoes.

Diet for Curing Cold Feet - Incorporate foods into your diet that generate warmth and induce blood flow. You should have plenty of beans, sprouted legumes*, Brussels sprouts, pumpkins, avocado, and spinach. All these are rich in antioxidants and vitamin E, and help promote a good circulation of blood.

Also, drink plenty of water, fresh fruit juices, and vegetable juices. Apples, oranges, apricots, grapes, plums, and cherries are rich sources of vitamin C and other healthy nutrients. Include a lot of heat-producing spices like anise, black pepper, caraway, cloves, cinnamon, ginger, and chilies in your diet to keep yourself naturally warm and healthy.

PROBLEM 11:   CORNS

Corns are a common foot problem, that usually occur as a result of wearing ill-fitting shoes for a prolonged time. When your shoes are uncomfortable and tight, they rub and press over certain areas of your foot. The skin then becomes hard and thick, forming an irregular thick growth called a corn.

Sometimes, the affected area becomes very painful, and infection may set in due to repeated irritation. In this case, surgical removal of the corn is an effective option. However, surgery is the last option in these cases, because early treatment of corns is adequate to control them and even remove them. Natural remedies for corns are both effective and safe.

I have listed below some important guidelines on corn care, along with natural remedies to treat corns effectively.

No More Ill-Fitting Shoes - The first and foremost step in the treatment of corns is to swear off ill-fitting footwear. Take pity on your feet and fling all those unnecessary and inefficient pairs of footwear from your closet—all the shoes that make your feet hurt when you wear them. Instead, shop for comfortable and elegant shoes that take the strain off your feet. Shop for comfort, not just style. Your shoes should have a toe area wide enough that you can wiggle your toes freely.

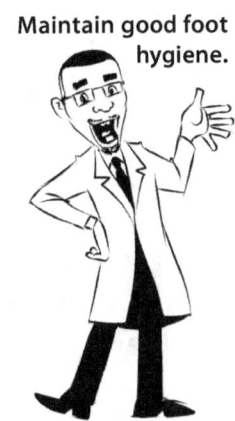

Maintain good foot hygiene.

Regular Scrubbing – A wonderful way to take care of corns is to use a pumice stone to scrub off dead skin from your feet every day. Take care not to scrub too vigorously, as you could damage healthy skin, resulting in a painful ulcer. You would probably find it easier to first soak your feet in warm water for some time. The dead skin absorbs water and softens, making it much easier to scrub it off gently.

Moisturize Regularly – Once your feet are clean and dry, moisturize them with a good moisturizer. This will ensure the corn doesn't dry out and the affected area heals faster. Castor oil is another excellent remedy for corns, as it penetrates into the deeper skin layers, softening them and making exfoliation* a breeze.

Soda Mix - Try applying a paste of baking soda, water, and lime juice over your corns at bedtime for a week. This is another very effective way to remove corns.

Chamomile Tea - Chamomile tea is also very helpful in healing corns. Mix some in a tub of hot water and indulge yourself in a thirty-minute hot water foot soak. This amazing herb is excellent at both healing sore corns as well as soothing your feet.

Kitchen Vinegar - A home-based ingredient that helps soften corns is ordinary vinegar. Place a cotton swab soaked in vinegar over the corn overnight. In the morning, just scrub the area gently with a pumice stone and wash. Pat your feet dry and apply a good moisturizer.

Papaya – Papaya is an incredibly effective antiseptic and healing fruit. It is usually mashed and applied on the corn overnight to soften it. Then debride the thickened skin with a pumice stone, to leave the area smooth.

PROBLEM 12:   CRACKED HEELS

Cracked heels are an extremely common problem and mostly reflect the neglect of proper foot care. In our busy schedules, we are often left with little time to care for our feet as they deserve. Months of such neglect result in painful and uncomfortable cracks developing in the heel area. Cracks mainly occur when the skin dries out. Thus, cracks are much more pronounced in the cold dry winter months than during summer. A regular foot moisturizing routine is essential if you want to avoid cracks.

These cracks and fissures in our heels can become very painful if not treated at an early stage. Since our feet bear the whole weight of the body, the pressure on our heels tends to deepen these fissures, potentially making them more serious. Moreover, an open wound may make your feet more susceptible to bacterial or yeast infections and can make your foot problems much worse.

Prevention and Remedial Measures

It is advisable to treat cracked feet and fissures as soon as they start developing to prevent the occurrence of more harm. The following pointers will help preserve, treat, and protect the health of your heel skin naturally at home.

Regular Pedicures – Pedicures are simple treatments, but you simply cannot afford to ignore them if you want to keep heel cracks at bay. A home pedicure consists of giving your feet a good soak in warm water with a mild soap, followed by gently scrubbing off the dead skin with a pumice stone. You will be astonished at the results you obtain. The warm soak softens the dead skin layers, making them easier to peel off, while the pumice stone scrub exfoliates the dead cells and the accumulated dirt. Giving your feet a regular pedicure will allow your heel skin to breathe freely and remain healthy, without the pores being blocked by dead cells and dirt.

Avoid Extreme Climates – You should take great care to protect your feet from exposure to biting cold during the winter. You should opt to wear good socks to protect your skin. Wash your feet regularly with warm water, but make sure not to go to the opposite extreme and use water that is too hot. It will strip your skin of its essential natural oils and dry it out still more.

Good Moisturizers – The use of a good moisturizing cream on the feet is another essential step in conditioning your feet and keeping the heels soft and supple. Olive oil, shea butter cream or jojoba are excellent moisturizers for the feet, and there are many other options. Whichever you choose, remember to apply it at least three times a day, and put on socks if you are going out or before you go to bed.

Foot Bath – If you have heel cracks and fissures, try using the hot and cold foot bath technique for truly amazing results. This consists of soaking your feet in hot and cold water consecutively a number of times. The variation in temperature stimulates foot circulation and hastens the healing of any existing cracks or fissures. If you can, add a few drops of an essential oil like lavender, tea tree, or cinnamon to boost the antibacterial effect of the hot water. The oils also soothe the skin and help heal bruises.

Wear Padded Shoes – Always remember to wear comfortable padded shoes when your heels are cracked to provide your feet with both comfort and support during this phase. You should never ever walk barefooted with cracked heels, because bacteria or fungi can easily gain access. Also, keep away from public showers, swimming pools, or gym locker areas until your feet are whole again, since these places provide ideal conditions for breeding fungi.

PROBLEM 13:   DRY FEET

Skin can dry out for several reasons. Some of the common causes are excessively dry climates, dietary deficiency of vitamins essential for skin health, the presence of fungal or bacterial infections, or other skin conditions. However, dry feet are easy to treat at home with the following tried and tested natural remedies.

Natural Remedies for Dry Feet

Stay Hydrated – Water is the most essential part of our bodies, not only cleaning and detoxifying the various body systems, but also keeping the tissues in a proper state of hydration. It is one of the very best natural moisturizers available. If you are properly hydrated, your skin will glow naturally, and many skin problems will be greatly lessened. Water is the natural antidote for dryness.

Vinegar Mix – If your feet are uncomfortably dry, add a little distilled white

Put sunblock on your feet while wearing

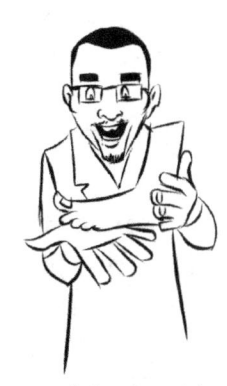

sandals to avoid sunburn.

35

vinegar to some warm water in a tub and soak your feet for at least half an hour once a week. This is effective in reducing foot dryness.

Essential Oils – Essential oils are among the greatest boon of Mother Nature. They include oils like tea tree, lavender, clove, olive, and coconut, which are all excellent moisturizers for your dry feet. Their deep moisturizing action means the oils seep through thousands of skin pores to soften skin deep down. Their potent antibacterial properties make sure that minimal bacteria can grow on the skin covering your feet. You need to make sure you are using pure organic essential oils to derive the greatest benefits. Use them daily on your feet and watch your skin becoming soft and flexible in front of your eyes!

Skin Pack – You can easily make up a foot scrub using rice powder, honey, and apple cider vinegar. Apply the pack to your feet with gentle rubbing. The pack will both exfoliate and moisturize your skin deep below the surface. In addition, apple cider and honey are known for their antibacterial properties.

Moisturizing Oil Mix – Make your own moisturizing mix with olive oil and almond oil. Rub this mixture gently on your feet every day using a cotton ball or your bare hands, so that the oils can seep down into your skin through the pores. This is an effective treatment for dry skin and cracked heels.

Include Vitamins in Your Diet - Vitamins like A and C are great skin health boosters, because they provide rich nourishment for the skin cells while restoring the natural oil balance of your skin. Fish oils like cod liver oil are rich sources of vitamin A. Citrus fruits and fresh green veggies yield plenty of vitamin C. Be sure to include these as much as possible in your daily diet.

PROBLEM 14:   FLAT FEET

Flat feet are usually the result of an inborn failure to develop a normal arch structure at the base of the feet. The absence of a foot arch is normal in infancy. However, the arch starts to develop around the time a child begins to walk, and continues to deepen till adulthood. In some people, this process is arrested for various reasons, resulting in flat feet.

The physical basis of flat feet is the malalignment of the ankle bones toward the mid-foot section. This causes an awkward gait and a tendency to lose one's balance. It is usually painless and not associated with any other complications. However, if it is accompanied by pain in the ankles, feet, or toes, it should not be ignored, as the pain could very well signal internal injury or inflammation of the arch area. This could involve the tendons in the posterior part of the foot. Medically, such a syndrome is termed "painful progressive flatfoot".

Treatment

A simple flat foot does not need treatment, but your footwear should be adjusted to compensate for the lack of an arch. If you have painful progressive flatfoot, you will require surgery, medications, physical therapy, and orthotics for treatment.

Acupressure*and foot massaging, like rolling foot the foot over circular objects like a tennis ball. Massaging devices hand held or foot spas are also proven to help flat feet. These help to relax the feet, also as an added benefit improves blood circulation. Flexibility of feet can be improved giving you better body alignment and toning. Acupressure is one of the best flat foot remedies as it is painless and relaxing. These natural suggestions will help by easing the tension of muscles.

PROBLEM 15:   **FOOT ODOR**

Foot odor is another very common complaint. It is also a very unpleasant and frustrating experience, since it disgusts others as well. This chapter explores the problems associated with and the remedies available for foot odor.

What Causes Foot Odor?

The medical term for foot odor is "bromhidrosis". Foot odor is due to bacteria breeding in the moist and humid conditions provided by sweaty feet and socks. Did you know that the soles of your feet have almost a thousand sweat pores that shed about a half cup of perspiration every day? This sweat is made up mostly of water, fat, sodium chloride, minerals, and acids, which represent waste products of the body.

The accumulated sweat acts as an ideal breeding ground for bacteria, which break down the secretions. This process involves the release of odorous by-products that contribute to that familiar odor of sweaty feet. There are simple but effective home remedies for this annoying condition.

Regular Cleansing – Keeping your feet clean by cleansing and washing them is one of the most important steps toward avoiding and treating foot odor. Wash your feet with a mild antibacterial soap to remove the smell-producing bacteria.

Rinse off the soap with warm water, rather than cold, since the heat opens the pores and cleanses the skin thoroughly. Pamper your feet with a thorough warm water soak once or twice a week to prevent foot odor from developing. If your feet already have odor issues, you will need to follow the daily routine of washing and rinsing as previously outlined. However, don't obsess about this! Too much washing can damage your skin still more.

Use Kosher Salt* - Kosher salt is an immensely effective natural sweat absorbent. If you have excessively sweaty feet, you could dissolve about half a cup of this salt in a quart of water and soak your feet in the solution for some time. Afterwards, dab your feet dry with a clean towel, without rinsing them. You will be astounded by the results. Your feet will remain naturally dry because the salt has a drying effect on the skin. This way, you can control your perspiration naturally to a large extent without any side effects. However, if you plan to do this, you must first make sure that you do not have any open wounds, cuts, or skin inflammation on your feet, since the salt could corrode them, leading to more damage.

Cut toenails straight across.

Wear Healthy Fabric – It is always best to wear socks made from light natural fabrics* like cotton and wool. These are both comfortable and breathable. However, you may prefer to choose from the array of other fabrics available, including rayon*, nylon*, and acrylic*. In that case, you should be careful to select those that suit the needs of your feet. Lighter materials are always better for sweaty feet, as they allow the free passage of air and thus keep your feet dry and clean.

Avoid tight socks because they can restrict circulation in your feet, making them cramp and sweat even more. Make it a practice to pick out fresh, clean socks every night for use the next day, while tossing your old socks into the laundry. This will make you feel happier, smell better and be way more comfortable.

Shoes - If you have sweaty feet, it is important that you choose footwear for summer that is open and allows free ventilation, so that your feet can breathe. This includes sandals, slippers, flip-flops, and floaters. All of these allow sweat to evaporate so that your feet remain dry, thus curbing bacterial growth on your feet.

However, if you prefer closed shoes, opt for canvas and leather shoes because they allow some air to pass through. For those with a high number of sweat pores on their feet, synthetic hard rubber footwear is an absolute no-no. If you use sneakers or canvas shoes, make sure you wash them at least once a week and let the air naturally dry them. This will keep your shoes clean and also inhibit microbial growth inside them.

If moisture is trapped inside your shoes, try dusting some baking soda or cornstarch powder inside them. This will absorb the moisture and prevent microbes from growing.

De-Stress - Stress is an important factor in the genesis of heavy perspiration. Anxiety disorders can lead to excessive sweating and a resulting offensive odor both from the body and feet. You need to practice a stress-free lifestyle. Learn to use simple positive meditation, yoga*, or breathing techniques to defuse stress when you are in a tense situation. Releasing stress has immense benefits, not only in relaxing the tension in your mind and body but greatly improving your overall health as well.

PROBLEM 16: FOOT PAIN

Foot pain is another very prevalent foot problem affecting all kinds of people. It is due to overexertion of the foot and general stress. It usually attacks those who stand for long hours, especially if their footwear is not comfortable and supportive. This can precipitate severe muscle cramps and foot discomfort. If you are overweight, standing for a long time puts additional pressure on your feet. This can result in a variety of issues like poor circulation in the feet, the formation of blood clots in the legs, edema of the feet and legs, or inflammation. These are serious issues and should be addressed immediately by your doctor.

In order to relieve the problem of foot pain, you need to pay attention to the state of your feet before irreversible damage sets in. If you have major symptoms like sudden pain, edema, acute discoloration, or severe pain, see your doctor at once. For general pain due to overuse, or following a long, hard day's work, natural remedies are best. These include ingredients that are readily available around you in your home.

Home Remedies for Foot Pain

Rest Your Feet – It is obvious that the first and most important remedy for foot pain is to make sure your feet get adequate rest. Avoid standing for long hours. If you have a standing job, take breaks in between to sit down and stretch your feet. Or put one foot up on a footstool while you stand. This by itself can make a great difference in the circulation in your feet.

Foot Bath - After a long day at work, it is very important that you give your feet a boost. Since your feet bear the weight and strain of your body throughout the day, you need to give them a good soak in warm water with a few drops of any essential oil that appeals to you. This will ease the strain and reduce the tiredness in your feet. Finish off with a moisturizer to leave your feet looking and feeling wonderful and comfortable again.

Alternate Foot Bath – Alternating soaking your feet between very warm water and cold water is a proven method to boost foot circulation. Place very warm and cold water in two separate tubs and put your feet into each tub alternately for a few minutes each.

Massaging – Pamper and comfort your feet with a good massage. This will improve the blood flow, tone up the muscles of your feet, and relieve the pain in your heels and ankles. You could use essential oils for the massage to boost the beneficial effect. A massage by a massage therapist or a foot expert would work best, but you can do it yourself if you wish. Remember to work the muscles from the ball of the foot to the tips of the toes using long deep strokes for the best effect.

Cold Compresses - Ice packs or cold compresses are another great way to soothe painful muscle twitches and reduce swelling in your legs and feet. If your feet burn, apply a simple ice bag to ease the sting.

Exercise - Foot exercise is very important in maintaining the general health of your feet. One example of a foot exercise is stretching the feet, ankles, and calves. While sitting, you can keep your heel on the floor and flex the foot, pulling the tops of the toes back toward the ankle. You can use a towel or stretch band to add tension. This works out muscles in the feet and strengthens them, so they can handle strenuous activity better.

It also improves the blood flow and keeps the feet supple. You should always remember to wear properly designed exercise shoes so that your feet are well supported during exercise. This will help protect them against injuries and accidents.

Toenail Trimming – You need to trim your toenails regularly to improve your foot hygiene. When your nails are unkempt, they invite all kinds of illnesses like fungal infections and ingrown toenails. Keep your nails short and clean, file the edges - especially around the corners - and finally, clean them gently with a nail file.

The Right Footwear – The wrong type of footwear can create many problems for your feet. Always choose comfort over fashion while selecting footwear to keep your feet healthy. Uncomfortable and ill-fitting shoes or sandals can cause serious foot damage and permanently impact your health at a later stage. Your shoes should support your foot structure, be made of flexible and soft materials, and allow your feet to breathe. A lot of thought should go into buying a pair of shoes!

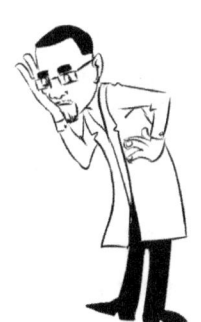

Don't ignore foot pain!

Proper Diet - Since feet are so important to us, it is essential to look after their nutritional needs. If you have puffy feet, you need to know that acidic foods or a high-salt diet can aggravate the swelling. Cutting these foods out of your diet can give you much relief. Too low a level of potassium* in your diet can also cause foot swelling, so include fruits like bananas with a high potassium content. Have ample servings of fresh fruits and vegetables, and plenty of water. This alone will flush out many of the toxins from your body. If your feet are prone to bacterial infections, try having foods like yogurt, and those which are rich in omega-3 fatty acids*, such as fish. These are potent antibacterial fighters.

Avoid Caffeine – Cut out caffeinated drinks like coffee and tea to avoid bloating or swelling of the feet. Instead, treat yourself to herbal teas and fresh fruit juices, which provide plenty of antioxidants and keep you glowing and healthy.

PROBLEM 17:   GOUT

Gout results from the buildup of uric acid* in the blood. Uric acid is the result of the breakdown of substances called purines* in the body. Usually it is dissolved in the blood, processed by the kidneys, and passed out of the body in the urine. But some people produce an excess amount of uric acid for various reasons. When there's too much for the kidneys to eliminate quickly, it builds up in the blood and seeps out into the tissues. There it may crystallize and collect in the joint spaces. This brings on the symptoms.

Gout symptoms come on quickly the first time, often overnight. You can go to bed feeling fine and wake up in excruciating pain. You may also have joint swelling with shiny red or purple skin around the joint. If you're already predisposed to gout, you can trigger an episode by:

- Drinking too much alcohol, especially beer
- Eating purine rich foods like red meats, animal organs, and fish
- Experiencing a sudden illness or trauma
- Going on a crash diet

Natural Treatments
Apple Cider Vinegar

Apple cider vinegar, which is used to treat headaches and acid stomach, also helps treat gout and arthritis. The acidity in apple cider vinegar will help relieve acute pain. You can also add honey to the remedy to boost the body's anti-inflammatory response.

- Mix one teaspoon of apple cider vinegar in a glass of water and drink it two to three times daily. If you find this remedy helpful, you can increase the dosage of apple cider vinegar to up to two tablespoons.
- Another option is to mix two tablespoons of apple cider vinegar with two tablespoons of honey. Take it two times daily, once in the morning and once before going to bed.

Ginger Root

The anti-inflammatory properties present in ginger root can be very helpful in relieving pain and inflammation. There are many ways to use ginger root in the treatment of gout.

- Mix equal amounts of fenugreek* powder, turmeric powder, and ginger root powder. Mix one teaspoon of this mixture with warm water. Take it twice daily.
- You can simply add grated ginger root into suitable recipes, or eat a small, raw piece of ginger root daily.
- You can also add one-half teaspoon of ginger root to one cup of boiling water and mix it well. Drink this solution at least once daily.
- Another option is to make a paste of ginger root with a little water and apply this paste on the affected area. Leave it on for about half an hour. Do this once daily.

Baking Soda

One significant factor contributing to gout is an increase of uric acid in the body. As an alkali, baking soda can help lower the amount of uric acid, giving you relief from the pain.

1. Mix one-half teaspoon of baking soda in a glass of water and drink it.
2. Drink this solution up to four times a day.
3. Continue up to two weeks.

If you are above 60 years old, do not take this more than three times in a day. Also, if you suffer from hypertension*, this remedy is not safe for you, as it increases the sodium* content of your body and, therefore, your blood pressure.

Lemon Juice

Fresh lemon juice and baking soda change the pH of the blood. Along with lemon juice, also eat other fruits rich in vitamin C to strengthen body tissues.

- Mix the juice of one lemon with one-half teaspoon of baking soda. Let it sit for a few seconds, and then mix it in a glass of water. Drink it immediately.
- Another option is to add the juice of half a lemon to a glass of water and drink it three times a day.

Pure Cherry Juice or Cherries

Cherries, whether sweet or sour, are rich in antioxidants* and can be very helpful in treating gout. Cherries also contain anthocyanins*, which can reduce inflammation as well as minimize gout flare-ups.

One 8oz daily glass of 100% cherry juice has been proven to reduce uric acid levels in the blood. This translates into a 30-40% reduction in gout pain.

Eating 15 to 20 cherries a day is highly recommended. For better results, eat them the first thing in the morning. Fresh cherries are best, but if they are not available at the market, you can opt for canned cherries.

Epsom Salts

Epsom salts are also useful in the home treatment of gout and other forms of arthritis. Add two cups of Epsom salts to a warm foot bath and soak your foot once a day as long as you have symptoms. The salt relaxes aching muscles and relieves pain from gout.

PROBLEM 18: HAGLUND'S DEFORMITY

(PUMP* BUMP)

Haglund's deformity is a painful swelling or lump on the back of the heel bone. It is more common in women than men, and is associated with the prolonged wearing of high-heeled shoes. The symptoms associated with this disorder include heel swelling, redness, soreness, and intense pain.

Treatment

If you suffer from this condition, it is best to avoid wearing high-heeled shoes. Comfortable flat shoes will relieve the pressure and stress on your heels. Try to find a pair with arch supports and cushion. Natural home-based remedies like warm herbal foot soaks, massaging with essential oils that have anti-inflammatory properties, and foot exercises are all useful in pain relief.

PROBLEM 19:   **HAMMERTOES**

Hammer toe is a foot deformity that is caused when the toe is permanently bent at its middle joint (PIPJ, proximal interphalangeal joint), making the toe look like a hammer. It is most common in the second, third, and fourth toes of the feet.

What Causes Hammer Toe?

Hammer toe is caused by the prolonged use of ill-fitting shoes that leads to uneven muscle stress in the feet. Genetics can be a factor as well, meaning you could conceivably blame this on your parents! Hammer toe can lead to the formation of other foot problems like corns, calluses, and blisters over the protruding middle joints or the tips of the toes. This results in pain and discomfort.

Treatment

Hammer toe should be treated at an early stage to prevent other foot complications from developing. Use footwear with wide, high forefoot space. This prevents your toes from having to scrunch up, keeping them from being irritated by the underside of the shoe. They will also be able to spread out freely, which helps distribute your body weight evenly.

To deal with pain in your feet and toes, you can soak your feet in warm water with a few drops of anti-inflammatory essential oils like lavender, eucalyptus, or peppermint oil. Use gel pads* or gel caps* over the bent toes to keep them from rubbing against the shoe. Exercise and stretch your feet regularly to strengthen your muscles and keep them more flexible. Wear shoes that are soft and have roomy toe boxes to keep the affected toe comfortable.

Inspect your feet regularly.

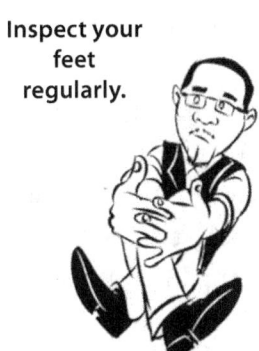

Pay attention to changes in color, texture or appearance.

PROBLEM 20: **HEEL PAIN**

Heel pain is a foot problem that millions of people struggle with. Its medical name is "plantar fasciitis". If your heel becomes painful when you sit for long periods, or after a good night's sleep - even though you can't recall any injury or trauma - your plantar fascia is usually the

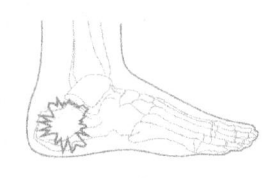

issue. This strange-sounding thing is a band of strong fibrous tissue stretching over the bottom of your foot. When it becomes inflamed, we call it plantar fasciitis. Also called heel pain, this condition is often accompanied by a heel spur*. The spur has exactly the same symptoms. However, it is not always present in every case of heel pain. A heel spur is a bony growth, while plantar fascia is a thickening of the ligamentous band that is inflamed at the bottom of the heel. Stretching of the arch can cause significant discomfort.

What are the Causes?

Plantar fasciitis is due to an inflammation of the plantar tissues, i.e. the bottom of the foot between the heel and toes. It manifests as severe pain in the heels, especially in the morning. If this is not attended to in time, it may become chronic and seriously impair foot function.

Heel pain can have many causes. It may affect all ages, from children to adults. The chief reason for an inflamed condition of the fascia is the excessive wear and tear that the foot goes through. This stress could be in the form of uncomfortable and ill-fitting shoes, high heels, foot deformity, increased activity, weight gain, weight loss, or simply prolonged strain on the feet.

Natural Remedies

Cold Compression - Cold compression with an ice pack is one of the best ways to reduce inflammation of the tissues. Use a daily ice pack wrapped in a towel on the painful area of your heel for visible results. Another method is to roll your feet on frozen or chilled bottles of water. This will result in your heels feeling far more comfortable. Also, roll a frozen lemon under your arch, this stretches the ligament and helps with the pain. If you don't have a lemon you can use a small ball.

Nothing Uncomfortable - Avoid wearing uncomfortable footwear such as tight shoes and high heels. This may aggravate the problem further by putting great strain on your heels and ankles. Instead, wear orthopedic pads and comfortable footwear that keeps your heels rested and in an even position.

Control Body Weight - It is essential to maintain a body weight on the lower end of the scale. The feet carry the weight of the entire body, with the brunt being borne by the heels. If you are overweight, your heels have to endure prolonged pressure and strain because of the excessive weight. The best way to prevent this and to provide relief to your heels is to maintain an ideal body weight.

Stretch The Ligament - Exercise is a very important factor in the healing of this kind of strain. You need to do gentle stretching exercises of the feet and legs. This will help reduce the pain of the plantar fascia. For example, as soon as you wake up, sit up and point your toes towards your nose. Hold for 15-20 seconds. You can use a towel or a stretch band to help. Calf raises are also good while standing. Eventually the pain should disappear.

Arch Supports – Your foot doctor can supply these. They help reduce the stress on the foot arches, and will support the foot and ankle.

PROBLEM 21:   **INGROWING TOENAILS**

An ingrown toenail is when a toenail cuts into the surface of the nearby skin. This common condition mostly affects the big toes.

What Causes an Ingrown Toenail?

Ingrown toenails occur when the nails are not cut evenly. This leads to irregular growth of the nails. They grow deep into the skin at the side of the nail, injuring it and causing a lot of pain.

Natural Treatment and Prevention

Ingrown toenails are curable and can be effectively controlled. Preventive measures include trimming your toenails straight across. The level of the nails should be the same as the tip of the toe. The sharp edges around the corners of the toenail should be filed so they cannot cut into the flesh at the sides of the nail bed.

If you already have an ingrown toenail, try applying geranium oil to the painful area. Geranium oil is a powerful antiseptic with healing properties and will speed up the healing of the affected area.

If your toenail has grown too deep into your flesh and you are unable to remove the ingrown nail by yourself, you will need to visit a podiatrist as early as you can. The doctor will remove the nail surgically. The skin and underlying tissue will then heal properly. However, cover the area with socks and wear shoes when you go out or are at work to protect the open nail bed from infection.

PROBLEM 22:   **MALLET TOE**

Mallet toe is basically a contracted toe condition. It is just like a hammer toe except that the joint affected is the DIPJ (**distal** interphalangeal joint), while hammer toe is a deformity of the PIPJ (**proximal** interphalangeal* joint). In general, they are perceived as identical.

This deformity occurs when the last joint (DIPJ) in the affected toe is unable to straighten. The deformed toe is forced to rub against the underside of the footwear. This continuous friction leads to pain and the development of other foot problems like corns and blisters.

Mallet toe usually affects poorly functioning joints of the toes, but can also result from prolonged arthritis of the toes. It can affect the normal functioning of your feet because of the significant pain and discomfort. If your footwear is not comfortable and well-fitting, it could worsen your condition and even impair your mobility.

Remedy and Prevention for Mallet Toe

To prevent mallet toe from affecting your foot function, take care of the problem at the very outset. Be aware of how your deformed toe is shaped, so you can predict which areas will be sensitive and take precautions to avoid injuring them. If it is overlooked, the condition could progress to more severe tissue damage and serious foot infection.

Proper shoes – If you have mallet toe, you should aim at shifting pressure and friction away from the sensitive areas and keep them as free as possible. This will ease the rubbing and irritation caused by your shoes. Select shoes that have a wide and high forefoot so that your toes have enough space for comfort. This will prevent corns, blisters, and other forms of friction foot injuries from developing in the mallet toe area.

Herbal footbath - If you have foot pain, blisters, corns, or other inflammation because of a mallet toe, give your feet a herbal footbath with fragrant essential oils like eucalyptus, lavender, peppermint, or bergamot oils. You can also massage them into the affected area.

In addition to these remedies, you can also wear gel toe caps or toe crests* on the affected area to protect it from further friction against your shoes. Gel caps will provide comfort, support, and soft padding to your toes, giving you immense relief from the discomfort and irritation caused by this deformity.

PROBLEM 23: METATARSALGIA

As the name implies, "metatarsalgia" is usually a painful foot condition that occurs due to sprain or pressure in the area between the arch and the balls of the foot. This pain usually occurs in the mid-foot area, where the ball of the foot is, and where the five metatarsal bones are in contact with the ground.

Metatarsalgia* is mainly due to obesity and overweight conditions, which make for an enormous amount of pressure in the mid-foot region. An injury to the foot could also cause inflammation of the metatarsal joints. Such injuries may be caused by sports, accidents, over-exercising, improper footwear, and walking on hard surfaces. Arthritis is another reason for this foot problem. Prolonged metatarsalgia can lead to callus formation on the underside of your feet.

Natural Treatment

The first and foremost treatment to reduce discomfort is to maintain an ideal body weight to avoid excessive pressure on the mid-section and front area of your feet. In addition, you should select good shoes with comfortable and sturdy heel support. Thirdly, soak your feet in warm herbal footbaths and massage your feet with essential oils for fast pain relief.

PROBLEM 24:   **PLANTAR FIBROMAS**

Plantar fibromas* are non-malignant lumps or tumors that grow inside a fibrous band in the foot, called the plantar fascia. These growths can cause pressure and foot pain, as well as lead to other more serious foot conditions.

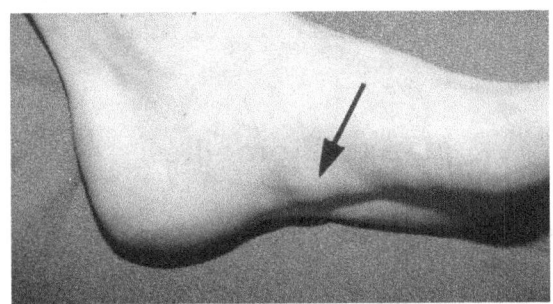

Treatment

These tumors* are difficult to treat with natural remedies. If they are surgically removed, they often grow back. The best way to deal with them is to adjust your footwear to compensate for their presence. Also, make allowance for the decreased pressure of your feet by limiting the strain you put on them. Give your feet as much rest as you can.

PROBLEM 25:   PLANTAR WARTS

A plantar wart is a viral infection that is caused by the "Human Papilloma Virus" (HPV). This wart appears as a small irregular bump on the sole of the foot. The virus is usually contracted through direct contact with another viral wart. The wart mostly affects the feet, but can also appear on other parts of the body due to its contagious nature.

Symptoms

Infection with this virus causes small blackish warts or lumps to appear on the surface of the sole. It is very itchy and also causes a lot of pain. The affected skin gradually becomes hard and thick as the wart enlarges, making walking painful.

Natural Remedies

1. Avoid scratching the affected area with bare fingernails; the virus can lodge under your nails and be spread to other parts of the body.
2. Always keep your feet dry and dust herbal antibacterial powders on the affected area regularly. The best powders for this use are those made from herbs such as sage, thyme, garlic, cedar, and pine.
3. Applying pure herbal remedies such as tea tree oil, turmeric, or cinnamon also help.
4. Always wear clean and fresh socks. Wash your socks well and let them air dry thoroughly before use. Do the same for your shoes. Let your shoes be exposed to the sunlight

or the open air for a while so the sweat and moisture inside dries completely. A very sensible yet hygienic option would be to wear alternate pairs of shoes so that each pair gets at least a day to dry.

The warts may take some time to disappear completely. However, if at any time the symptoms become more severe, you need to get medical help from a podiatrist.

PROBLEM 26:   PREGNANCY

Foot Problems Related to Pregnancy

Pregnancy causes many changes to occur in a woman's body. These changes are natural and common. Foot pain is one such issue. The usual reason is the natural increase in weight during pregnancy that causes sudden extra strain and pressure on the feet. The increased strain in turn causes foot problems, most commonly, flat feet or over-pronation,* and edema.

Don't hide ugly toenails with polish.

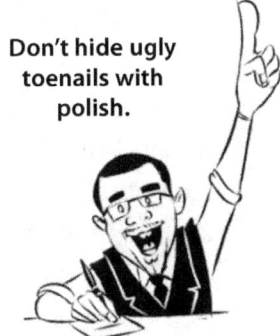

See your podiatrist.

Both these problems cause similar symptoms like pain in the heel and ball of the foot, pain in the arch area, swollen feet, mild to severe leg cramps, and, in some cases, varicose veins. But taking care of your feet during pregnancy can help avoid serious foot problems.

How do Edema and Over-Pronation Affect the Feet?

Edema or swelling of the feet is more typical in the latter half of pregnancy. The reasons behind it are many. One is that the volume of circulating blood increases during pregnancy. Another is that the increase in size of the uterus makes it a large and bulky organ. It compresses the veins which return blood from the lower parts of the body, that is, the pelvis and legs. This results in slow circulation. Fluid under increased pressure seeps out of the blood vessels in the legs and feet, manifesting as edema. A third reason is that salt and water are retained in excess during pregnancy. This shows up as excessive fluid outside the blood vessels, in the soft tissues of the feet, which causes swelling and discomfort. In a few cases, the feet show a dark purplish discoloration.

If you are pregnant, you need to make sure there is no swelling in any other part of the body, for instance, in the neck, face, or hands. If this occurs, you will need to consult your gynecologist immediately.

Over-pronation of the feet leads to a flat-footed walk in late pregnancy. This is again mostly due to excess weight. The added burden on the feet causes flattening of the natural arch. The band of fibrous tissue stretching from the back to the front of the heel becomes overstretched. Finally, it becomes inflamed and painful, which makes walking very uncomfortable

Treatment and Prevention

There are many natural home-based remedies for treating both edema and flat feet syndromes. The first and most important measure is to choose comfortable and padded footwear to protect and support your feet properly. There are many specially designed shoes available to treat such feet problems. If you suffer from flat feet, make sure your footwear gives good arch support for your feet. If your feet are swollen, use footwear with ample toe boxes. Wearing shoes that are too tight can restrict the blood flow in your feet and increase the pain and swelling.

The next step in edema of the feet is to elevate your feet as high as you comfortably can, whenever possible. For example, while sitting, you could rest them on a stool in an easy position.

Also, use cold compresses regularly on your feet. Placing your feet under running cold water is one way to apply cold compresses. You can also try soaking your feet in a solution of baking soda, Epsom salts, and cold water.

Other treatments for edema include the following:

- Wear good quality loose and seamless socks to allow blood to circulate freely.
- Avoid strenuous activities.
- Take short breaks in the middle of your work to stretch your feet, as this will promote free circulation.
- Schedule light exercises like walking, which will be of great help in keeping you active and stress-free.
- Remember to keep yourself hydrated by drinking plenty of water, because this will decrease the amount of fluid you retain, or edema fluid.
- Have a balanced diet. Include a lot of antioxidant rich foods like fresh fruits, vegetables, and omega-3 fatty acids.
- Reduce the amount of salt in your food, since this tends to promote water retention.

Both feet are usually swollen to the same extent if you have edema. If one foot is much more swollen than the other, you need to consult your gynecologist. Keeping tabs on your health is vital in pregnancy to keep you and your child safe.

PROBLEM 27:   STIFF ANKLE

A stiff ankle can be caused by many things: rheumatoid arthritis, inflammation, or degenerative joint disease (DJD) i.e. arthritis. It can also be caused by an abrupt twisting or bending of the ankle joint, which results in putting too much stress on the ligaments. The cartilage, bone, or ligaments may be torn or inflamed. Constant stress on the joints can also cause them to stiffen over time, especially in athletes. Stiff ankles usually cause swelling, tenderness and pain, along with restricted ankle movement. X-rays and blood tests will be necessary to find out why your ankles are stiff. Many types of joint diseases can show these symptoms.

Treatment

Treating a stiff ankle requires that the foot be given sufficient rest. Cold compresses may reduce the swelling. Once the swelling has gone down, hot compresses will help reduce muscle stiffness.

Epsom Salts Bath – Add 1 tablespoon of salt to half a gallon of water. Soak your feet daily in this solution for 15-20 minute soaks to reduce the stiffness in the ankle. Peppermint and spearmint essential oils added to the bath can also help with relaxing the muscles.

In severe cases of stiff ankle, surgical intervention may be required to remove damaged cartilage or to repair ligaments and/ or tendons in the ankle.

| PROBLEM 28: | SWOLLEN FEET |

Puffy feet are another common problem. This condition is also known as edema. In many cases the feet look normal early in the morning, but they slowly swell over the day, making it difficult to put your shoes back on. The puffiness may be accompanied by pain, fatigue, and exhaustion.

Edema can be due to several medical conditions, which are often heralded by very subtle symptoms like tired and aching feet. Even in very serious conditions, the swelling may be minimal in the initial stages. This is why you should never ignore persistent puffiness, even if it is slight at first.

Stop! Consult your medical doctor!

The symptoms of edema may be easily overlooked at first. For instance, a previously comfortable pair of shoes may suddenly become curiously tight. Indentation marks around the ankle may appear from socks and last a long time. These may be warning signals for you to take action immediately.

Anyone can develop edema. In many cases it is due to over-vigorous foot activity or too much stress on your feet. In other cases, an exhausting journey, insomnia, or a high salt diet can result in edema. If you notice puffiness around the ankles, you may find it advisable to lower your sodium or salt intake since a high salt content in the blood tends to increase edema. However, edema by itself is not a very serious problem and can easily be treated naturally at home.

Use Comfortable Foot Wear - If you have puffy feet, wear loose and comfortable footwear. Take care to avoid wearing anything that puts strain on your feet, like ill-fitting shoes, raised heels, and platforms. Flat heels or even level foot wear are the best options for anyone who has edema, because they put no strain on the ankles. Ankle strain can increase tension in the structure of the foot, leading to swelling and pain. Be kind to your feet and choose to wear footwear that gives your swollen feet relief and comfort.

Alternate Foot Bath - Alternating hot and cold foot baths are another very effective method to alleviate swelling and improve blood circulation to your feet. This completely natural method is also one of the most effectual treatments for swollen feet. However, diabetics should never start a soaking treatment without consulting their doctor.

To give your feet alternate hot and cold baths, have two containers ready, one filled with hot water and the other with cold. Take two footbaths or basins and pour the water into them. Add water to adjust the temperatures of both hot and cold tubs to your comfort level so the footbath does not damage your skin.

Now seat yourself comfortably and immerse your feet for fifteen minutes at a time alternately in the hot and cold water. In between, you elevate your feet, placing them on a towel on top of a footstool for a few minutes. Continue this until you feel relief. Finish up with the hot water. Blot your feet dry with the towel. This treatment has been found to markedly reduce foot swelling and improve the circulation, providing immense comfort to puffy feet.

Watch Your Diet - Avoid very salty foods and limit your salt intake in general, as it may lead to water retention in the body. High sodium intake not only increases blood pressure, but also causes your feet to swell up and become bloated.

Also keep away from processed foods like frozen and packaged meals, canned soups, etc., that are high in sodium content.

In addition to these, it is important to drink plenty of water and keep your body hydrated. Adequate hydration leads to less water retention in the body overall and in your feet in particular.

Massage – A massage is another natural treatment for reducing edema in the feet. Of course, you could always massage your own feet but it's much better to get it done professionally. The massage encourages the pooled fluid outside the blood vessels to re-enter the circulation, so that it can be flushed out via the kidneys into the urine, and thus leave the body permanently.

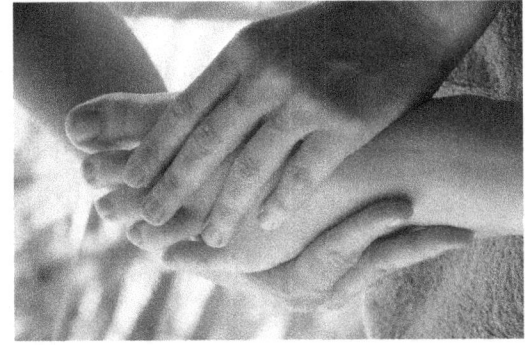

Herbal Cure – A variety of herbal treatments are available for puffy feet. Some of these, which are extremely effective in reducing foot swelling and making your feet feel young again, are listed below.

1. Blend lemon juice, water, milk, cinnamon, and olive oil in a bowl. Apply the mixture over your swollen feet and let it soak in for about 20 minutes. Rinse off and pat your feet dry.

2. Mix some baking soda and rice water in a container. Submerge your feet in the solution. Baking soda is an extremely good absorbent that soaks out excessive water from your feet through the skin pores, so the swelling is significantly reduced.

3. Another natural method of reducing the swelling of your feet is the popular "RICE" treatment. "RICE" stands for: Rest, Ice, Compression, and Elevation. Rest your foot by not putting weight on it for a while. Apply ice packs on the affected area. Continue this at intervals until the swelling subsides. Then wrap the foot using a compression bandage to a comfortable tightness. This should be kept on all the time, even when you walk. Keep your foot elevated whenever you sit down.

4. Ginger is a well-known anti-inflammatory herbal ingredient that can reduce painful swelling in the foot. Boil a generous amount of grated ginger in a pan with water. Pour the concoction into a tub and soak your feet in it. The relief you feel will be instant. There are other herbs like turmeric and Boswellia* that have similar properties and can be used in the same way. You can also infuse these herbs in your food and drink to obtain even greater benefits.

Eat Potassium-Rich Foods - Foods rich in potassium include soya flour, bananas, apricots, tomatoes and tomato products, sultanas, raisins, potatoes, figs, currants, avocados, beets, Brussels sprouts, cantaloupes, dried dates, kiwi fruit, lima beans, melons, nectarines pears, oranges, unsalted peanuts, prunes, spinach, and winter squash.

PROBLEM 29:   **TAILOR'S BUNION**

A tailor's bunion, also known as a bunionette, is a bump or prominence on your fifth metatarsal bone, at the base of your little toe. Your metatarsal bones are the five long, thin bones in your mid-foot that attach to your toes. Tailor's bunions are less common than regular bunions, these occur on the inside of your foot whereas tailor's bunions are on the outside of the foot.

Causes and Symptoms

Improperly fitting shoes is a main cause of tailor's bunions. The tapered toe boxes of most conventional shoes push your fifth toe toward your fourth toe, immobilizing your little toe in this deformed position. Your fifth toe, when it is held in this position, is more susceptible to trauma from your shoe. Most shoes available to consumers are not wide enough for the typical foot.

A tailor's bunion also may be caused by inherited. You will notice your fifth metatarsal bone begin to protrude on the outside aspect of your foot while your fifth toe shifts toward your foot's midline, creating a bump in this area that is irritated when your shoe rubs against it.

In some cases, it may be confused with a bone spur that is on the side of your fifth metatarsal head. It is actually a protrusion of bone.

A tailor's bunion causes the same symptoms as a regular bunion. Common signs and symptoms associated with a tailor's bunion include, pain, redness and swelling.

The symptoms are made worse by wearing shoes that have narrow toe boxes, which will rub against your bunionette and irritate the area including the underlying tissue.

Treatment

Most tailor's bunions can be treated by restoring the alignment of your foot bones. Some strategies for resolving this health problem include

- Avoid footwear that squeezes or pinches your forefoot. Choose shoes that possess a wide toe box and little or no heel elevation. See our shoe list for healthy footwear examples.
- Icing: Icing your affected area may reduce your pain and inflammation. Always wrap your ice pack in a thin towel when icing your problem area.
- Padding: Pads, especially bunionette pads, may help decrease your pain.

- Anti-inflammatory agents: Certain prescription drugs and dietary supplements may be helpful in reducing your bunion-related inflammation.
- Soaking in Epsom salt will help to calm the inflammation. Also add some essential oils for example peppermint oil, to soothe and relax the foot.

In some advanced cases as in all foot problems surgery may be needed.

PROBLEM 30:   TOE CRAMPS

Toe cramps* are also common and result from letting the toes remain in an uncomfortable or abnormal position for too long. This can occur with the use of ill-fitting footwear, dehydration, or strenuous exercise. You can recognize it by the feeling of pain and strain in the regions around the affected toe.

Natural Remedies for Toe Cramps

Why is the new dance called "The Elevator"? Because it has no steps!

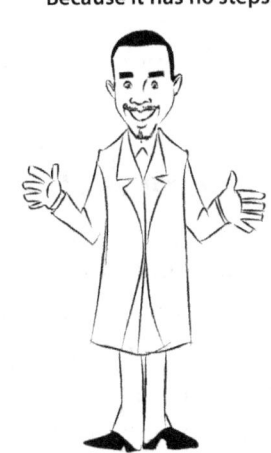

There are many ways to reduce toe cramps. Since they are typically caused by tight footwear, it makes sense to discard poorly fitting footwear and buy shoes that are both comfortable and spacious.

If your cramps follow a strenuous exercise regimen, you need to stop exercising and give your toes a gentle stretch in all directions to ease the pain. This is essential to prevent muscle tears. If you have severe pain, you should rest your feet until the level of pain goes down. You can hasten this process by soaking your feet in warm water with a few drops of eucalyptus or peppermint oil to relax them. This will not only soothe the feet but also encourage proper circulation.

PROBLEM 31:   TOENAIL FUNGUS

Toenail fungus is a very difficult condition that afflicts the toenails of the feet. Also called "onychomycosis" in medical parlance, it is quite common. It is due to infection by a class of fungi called dermatophytes, which are usually found in dark, soiled, and moist surroundings. It can often require repeated courses of treatment, and even then it may take a long time to be completely eradicated. The pain and rotting away of the nails often results in severe disability.

Please note that if your nails are very thick and dystrophic*, the following treatments will not help. Visit your local podiatrist for more effective treatments.

Symptoms of Toenail Fungus

With toenail fungus, the dermatophytes breed in the living tissue under the nails, making their home in the nail bed. The first sign of active infection is often the appearance of white or yellow spots under the nail as it gets separated from the underlying blood supply of the nail bed.

As the infection gradually spreads, the nail becomes thickened, crusty, and discolored. In the later stages, the color of the nail darkens; the nail is distorted and becomes brittle, often loosening from the nail bed. This can result in considerable pain and discomfort, mainly at the tips of the toes. Sometimes, the fungal infection is accompanied by a fetid odor.

What Causes Toenail Fungus?

Toenail fungus is most likely to be acquired in places that are warm, humid, and dark, like swimming pools, public showers and lockers, gym lockers, sweaty and moist shoes, instruments used during unhygienic pedicures, and washrooms. The infection is usually transmitted through an open cut or abrasion from a person afflicted with toenail fungus, or through their cast off brittle nail chips.

The fungus can affect anyone, especially those who have a weak immune system or immune deficiency. Diabetics, people who sweat too much, and those who have had athlete's foot before are susceptible to this problem. Poor blood circulation is an important contributing factor, which not only makes it difficult for the body to react to the fungal infection in time, but also impedes healing of the infection.

Natural Herbal Home Remedies for Toenail Fungus

Vinegar – This is an age-old antifungal agent. Soak some cotton wool with vinegar and apply it to the affected area as many times a day as you can. Or you could try taking a vinegar footbath using a mixture of two parts warm water and one part vinegar. A safe and effective method, its only drawback is that it might take up to a month to see visible results.

Essential Oils – Essential oils like tea tree, oregano, pine, cedar, and clove are very effectual remedies for toenail fungus. Paint these oils on your affected nail every day to see a rapid improvement in nail health and to keep the fungus at bay. Tea tree oil in particular has a strong antifungal and antibacterial action.

Homemade Anti-Fungal Ointment – Make your own potent antifungal ointment with the following ingredients: 1 cup of pure olive oil, half an ounce of any herbal powder mix containing at least three antifungal herbs (for example, basil, peppermint and thyme), and a few drops of tea tree oil or any other antibacterial oil of your choice. Lavender and coconut oil are two good examples. These herbal ingredients are easily available from any health store. Use this homemade ointment on the affected nail area at least twice a day to speed up the recovery of your nail.

Grapefruit Seed - Another natural ingredient for treating fungal infection is grapefruit seed extract. This oil is just as effective as tea tree oil with similar properties. Healing is generally seen within two months.

Garlic - Garlic is also a very effective antifungal spice. If you use it on the affected area, it can work wonders. You can either rub a clove of raw garlic on the toenail every day, or use it in ointment or powdered form. You could even try eating two or three cloves of raw garlic every day to deliver a boost to your immunity and speed up the healing process.

Olive Leaf Extract - This is another potent herbal agent for fighting toenail fungus. Olive leaf is a very strong natural antibiotic that fights all kinds of bacteria and fungi. It also cleanses and detoxifies the body by stimulating the immune system.

Precautions and Preventive Measures for Fighting Toenail Fungus

- Always trim your toenails straight across, keep them short, and clean and file them regularly.
- Disinfect your scissors, files, and nail cutter after every use to maintain hygiene.
- Avoid moist and dark areas and keep your feet dry (apart from when you are bathing).
- If possible, avoid public baths, wet swimming pool floors, and locker areas.
- For foot protection, always wear at least sandals or flip-flops; never walk barefooted in damp areas. Wear water-proof footwear to protect your feet from water.
- Change your socks and hose daily. Wear a fresh and clean pair every day. Women should try to avoid synthetic materials in particular since they block the free passage of air, resulting in increased sweat production.
- Air your shoes regularly in the sunlight to allow the moisture inside to dry out completely.
- Discard old exercise shoes, which can be a breeding place for fungi.
- Never borrow or wear other people's footwear, socks, towels, and other personal items, as they may transfer a fungal infection to you.

- Don't use cosmetics and nail paints on your toenails if they are infected, since nail paint can protect the infected area from air and allow the fungus to grow.
- Always dry your feet completely after a bath or wash.

If you are diabetic or suffering from immune deficiency, take extra care of your feet. A fungal infection could lead to serious foot complications, including possible amputation.

Chapter 3

Diabetes

iabetes mellitus is a serious disease that is characterized by the deficit of insulin production in the body. Insulin is an enzyme that is produced by the pancreas* to break down and process food components in our body into sustainable energy. The glitch occurs when there is a deficiency in the production of insulin or when the body is unable to use the insulin produced to properly process its food. When this phenomenon occurs, it leads to abnormally high glucose levels in the blood. This could lead to progressive and serious impairment of the immune system and many body organs, especially the eyes, kidneys, legs, and feet.

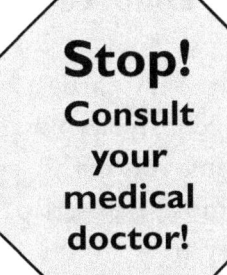

Stop!
Consult
your
medical
doctor!

Diabetes can be classified into two different types:

- Type 1
- Type 2

Type 1 diabetes is first seen in childhood and has a strong family tendency. Type 2 is the kind that manifests in adulthood. It is caused chiefly by obesity and a poorly controlled and unbalanced diet. Without proper control, it can cause serious health complications like nerve damage, glaucoma, and renal failure. It can also lead to cardiovascular disease.

As diabetes progresses, the nervous system - especially of the legs and feet - is the earliest to be affected. Though it is not curable, it can be well-controlled with proper discipline and care. It is extremely important to recognize the early symptoms of diabetes before complications set in. If you have already been diagnosed with diabetes, you need to keep a careful watch on your legs and feet. The following section deals with common foot problems in diabetes, their symptoms, and preventive measures. Hopefully, by the end of the section, you will have a clearer understanding of the importance of foot care for diabetics.

How Diabetes Affects Your Feet

In the very earliest stages of diabetes, your body's immunity is reduced. Thus, your ability to fight infection and illness decreases, making you highly susceptible to infections. Since your feet are the most exposed part of your body and are at greatest risk of injury, they are the first to be infected in most cases of diabetes.

Deterioration of the nervous system happens gradually after the onset of diabetes. This leads to your body becoming less receptive to touch and other physical sensations. Your feet may lose sensation and become numb. As sweat and oil glands slowly lose function, the skin over your foot becomes dry and hardened. The combination of these different effects of nerve damage cause undue pressure to be put on your foot skin. This is how foot sores and blisters form.

Since your immune system is already impaired, the body's ability to fight infections is affected. The healing process also takes much longer. This prolonged healing time increases the risk of other bacterial and fungal infections setting in and spreading, eventually leading to foot conditions like ulcers, non-healing wounds, circulation issues, and the risk of amputation. Therefore, care must be taken to prevent such foot infections.

It is very important for diabetic people to be fully aware from the very beginning that such problems are always lurking. You have to inspect your whole body every day to recognize the earliest signs of any damage. Modify your diet to keep your blood sugar within a normal range. Pay attention to your feet, looking for any wounds, calluses, or infections. Also make sure that sensation is normal in both feet from time to time. If you identify signs of nerve damage early, you can start treatment at once.

There have been enormous advances in the management of the diabetic foot. These help reduce pain and inflammation very efficiently, as well as promote complete healing. There are also many natural preventive measures and solutions for diabetic foot care, available within your home environment. However, the first step is to recognize the symptoms correctly.

Diabetic Foot Complications I

1. Constant foot pain may be the result of some unnoticed bruises, cuts, sprains, blisters, or other injury to your feet. Make sure they are not because of ill-fitting shoes. Check your feet thoroughly to locate the cause of your pain.

2. Inflammation or redness in any area of your feet might be caused by friction or abrasions from your socks and shoes. Remember, in diabetes these may or may not be painful.

3. Swollen feet may be caused by internal injury, infection, or inflammation caused by ill-fitting shoes or other external factors. Poor circulation of blood to your feet could also result in swelling. This swelling may be accompanied by symptoms like pain in the legs and hips, reduced hair growth over the legs, hardening of the skin, and difficulty in walking.

4. You might notice considerable warmth around an innocent looking wound that could signal the presence of internal inflammation or infection. This may persist for a long time, since healing is slow in diabetes. The wound may or may not heal with time.

5. Open wounds or breaks in the skin could prove to be very dangerous since such wounds could harbor microbes, either fungi or bacteria.

6. If you have a cut in the foot accompanied by fever and chills, seek medical advice at once! It could very well be a life-threatening infection. The fever and chills could be a sign of the spread of infection into the bloodstream.

7. Red streaks radiating from the area of the wound should be taken seriously, as this indicates the spreading of infection through the lymph vessels to the neighboring tissues. This could result in severe and deep foot infection.

8. If you don't have any visible wound or sign of infection in your feet but still have difficulty walking, then the problem area could be your joints and leg muscles.

9. Numbness of the feet is inevitable and progressive in diabetes. This makes it all the more essential that you increase the level of foot care as the years go by to minimize your risk of impairment.

Diabetic Foot Complications II

For people with diabetes, proper foot care is a very important step towards successful foot care management. High blood sugars often put people with diabetes at risk for neuropathy, or nerve damage. This can cause loss of sensation in the feet, leading to other serious complications such as ulcers, non-healing wounds, circulation issues, and the risk of amputation. Proper care will help you prevent these complications.

The foot of a diabetic is exposed to many injuries during day-to-day life. These foot injuries may result from external or internal factors. These can be carefully treated to prevent complications. Of the sixteen million Americans who suffer from diabetes, only 25% develop foot problems associated with the disease. This section discusses some of the significant risk factors that are intricately linked with diabetic foot injury.

Neuropathy – Diabetic neuropathy is a complication of diabetes that shows gradual progression and ultimately affects the functioning of the nervous system. This inevitably leads to diminished sensitivity in the legs due to nerve damage in the feet. This condition is called peripheral neuropathy, as it involves the nerves far away from the head and spine. It is an early complication of poorly controlled diabetes. However, if properly managed, its progression can be delayed.

The symptoms of neuropathy in the legs are the loss of normal sensations of heat, cold, and pain in the feet. This means the patient can no longer sense minor injuries like blisters, cuts, pressure sores, feet strain, corns, and calluses. These therefore go untreated and can develop into much more severe problems, even ending in amputation. Other less serious outcomes are chronic foot infections like toenail fungus, Charcot foot*, bunions, and warts. All this underlines how essential it is that a diabetic take daily stock of the state of his or her feet to prevent a lot of grief and pain later.

Poor Circulation – Peripheral vascular disease is another serious complication caused by diabetes. This is characterized by hardening and narrowing of the arteries, which is medically called atherosclerosis. The constricted and partially clogged arteries are unable to carry adequate oxygen-carrying blood to all parts of the body. Low oxygen levels lead to a less efficient healing process, causing foot complications like bacterial or fungal infections, ulcers, and gangrene. The feet can become dry and swollen.

Foot Infections – If you are diabetic and have any foot swelling or infection like athlete's foot, toenail fungus, calluses, ingrown toenails, and sores, you should seek immediate medical treatment. If you ignore foot symptoms and delay getting treatment, they may develop into serious infections that could be life threatening.

Diabetic Foot Natural Care & Prevention

A healthy lifestyle coupled with some preventive measures will help you deal with diabetic feet in a better way. Discussed below are some safe and natural diabetic foot care measures that will help you a great deal in managing this disease effectively.

Footwear – Selecting the right footwear is top priority when dealing with a diabetic. Your podiatrist or diabetes specialist would be able to recommend the right type of shoes that will be both comfortable and safe for your feet. Orthotic shoes are usually recommended for diabetic feet since such shoes are specially designed to protect them from heat, abrasion, and pressure. Whatever your decision, you should end up with shoes that have a wide and high space in the toe area and removable insoles to adjust heel pressure and flexibility.

Foot Examination – You should make it a point to examine your feet daily for any visible cuts, sores, swelling, redness, patches, or minor injuries. This process is vital and should be an integral part of your daily routine. This is extremely important because your feet have already lost a good deal of their normal sensitivity, so you may not be able to feel small injuries. Ask a family member to help you examine your feet all over if required.

Prompt Treatment – Any minor cuts or blisters that take more than two days to heal should receive prompt medical attention. Do not ignore the injury! It could give rise to serious complications. You can use natural home remedies to initially treat such infections. Essential oils like lavender, bergamot, and tea tree are very effective for treating such wounds. However, if the cut still refuses to heal, you need to see your physician as soon as possible.

Wash Your Feet Daily – Another extremely important measure for a diabetic is keeping your feet clean. Washing them with lukewarm water and a mild antibacterial soap every day is a great way to maintain the hygiene of your feet. Avoid using very hot water since it has a drying effect, stripping off the skin's natural oils. After washing your feet, dry them thoroughly and gently, especially between the toes. Follow this up by dusting some talcum powder over your feet to absorb any residual moisture.

Moisturize Your Feet – Moisturizing diabetic feet is a vital requirement, especially during the winter months. Since diabetic feet are naturally prone to dryness, moisturizing both the upper and the lower sides daily can be beneficial for the skin. However, do not rub lotion or cream between your toes.

Always Wear Shoes and Socks – Since diabetic feet are highly injury-prone, it is important to keep your feet covered and protected. Wearing shoes and socks prevents injury by external objects. But you should make it a point to first check the inside of your shoes thoroughly for any foreign objects like stone chips. This will keep your feet from getting hurt. Choose socks made from natural fabrics like cotton and wool, which help your feet breathe. Socks also help prevent the occurrence of painful sores and blisters. Avoid tight-fitting elastic socks and nylon hosiery, as they are notorious for impairing blood circulation. Choose comfortable shoes that provide protection to your feet.

Protection from Heat and Cold – Always protect your feet from exposure to hot or cold temperatures or objects. For example, never walk barefooted on beaches or pavement. Never keep diabetic feet uncovered or exposed. Keep away from fires, very hot water, heating pads, and radiators. Similarly, avoid exposing your feet to cold weather or snow. Wear thick padded socks during winter to protect your feet from frostbite. Always wear warm seamless socks at bedtime; sleeping barefooted during cold winter nights is dangerous.

Trim Your Toenails – Always trim your toenails with a proper nail clipper. Never use scissors or any other sharp objects to cut your nails, as these may cause injury. Cut the nails straight across and evenly. Do not cut your nails too close to the nail bed. Ask for help if you have difficulty trimming them. File the rough and sharp edges around the corners to prevent ingrown toenails. Diabetics must remember to keep regular appointments with their podiatrist to get their nails trimmed. This may sound unimportant, but this simple step can often save diabetics from potential amputations.

Be Active – Move your feet as much as possible. Mobility increases blood flow to your feet. If you have to sit for more than a few minutes, elevate your legs on a low stool. Keep rotating your ankles from side to side and wiggle your toes for a minute or two every now and then to keep the blood flowing while you are sitting. Change your position regularly. Shift your posture from time to time so that your feet are moving.

Exercise – Exercise works wonders for your feet. Regular exercise tones your joints and muscles and keeps your blood circulation healthy. Choose exercises that focus on improving blood circulation to your feet. Exercise also helps control blood sugar levels in your body. However, do not overexert yourself. This could cause muscle or ligament sprains and other injuries. Always wear good athletic footwear to protect your feet from injuries while working out. Cardiovascular exercises like swimming, brisk walking, and cycling are good for diabetic patients. Avoid jogging, running, and other high-impact exercises to prevent unnecessary pressure on your feet.

Quit Smoking – Smoking can tip the balance for diabetic patients. It could precipitate serious nerve and blood vessel damage. By quitting smoking, you will take a crucial step to preventing diabetic foot disease.

Control Your Sugar Level – This is the most important factor in managing this disease. Good glucose control can prevent a whole number of complications. For best results, follow a sensible diabetic diet, take proper medication, and check your blood sugar regularly. This will keep you in touch with your level of control and what modifications you need. Keep to a strict follow-up schedule with your physician and promptly report any new developments or problems. This will allow your physician to guide you properly and safely. Only strict diabetic control can lower your risk of damage to the legs, nervous system, kidneys, or eyes.

Maintain Weight – If you are diabetic and have foot disease, it is of the highest importance to maintain an ideal body weight. Obesity can produce severe pressure on your feet and leg joints, resulting in joint injuries and feet exhaustion. Weight reduction may be a challenging goal with diabetes, but it is definitely achievable with time and patience. There are many helpful weight-reducing diabetic diets that you can follow. Always ask your physician first to prevent any complications.

Observing these guidelines and precautions will make managing diabetes an easier task for you. Diabetes is a serious disease, but with a regulated and healthy lifestyle, you can manage it and live normally, without developing diabetic foot complications.

Please remember, the publication of this information does not constitute the practice of medicine, and this information does not replace the advice of your physician or other health care provider. Before undertaking any course of treatment, the reader should seek the advice of his or her physician or other health care provider.

Chapter 4

Foot Care Ingredients Found In Your Home

You may be surprised to know how many natural foot care ingredients you can find at home or your nearby store. Your kitchen has an array of beneficial herbs, spices, and natural ingredients that can alleviate many common feet ailments. Being aware of their properties and powers can arm you with health and vitality. Let us glance at the assorted herbs and natural ingredients that you can find in your kitchen to treat various common foot problems.

Spearmint Oil - Spearmint oil is a well-known essential oil that has valuable antiseptic properties. This is available in most households, yet it is used to cure many microbial infections. It is also used to soothe and heal insect bites, fungal and bacterial infections, indigestion, colitis, muscular injuries, throat and respiratory problems. It can be used as an oil or in the form of a cream. Spearmint oil is antiseptic, curative, and an excellent tonic for the skin.

What does a shoemaker use to repair shoes?

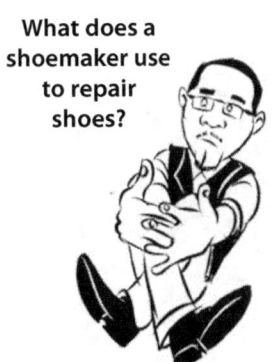

Toe-nails!

Epsom Salts - This widely used antifungal and antibacterial home-based ingredient is commonly used to treat fungal infections of the feet. Epsom salts contain the crystalline mineral magnesium sulfate. It is known for its soothing and exfoliating properties. It can relax the stressed muscles of the feet and is of great help in cleansing and purifying the skin. Simply soaking your feet in a tub of warm water mixed with a generous handful of Epsom salts will calm and soothe your feet.

Almond Oil - Light and subtle in fragrance, almond oil effectively treats dry skin. It is an essential oil that is used in many beauty products and is known for its nutritional benefits.

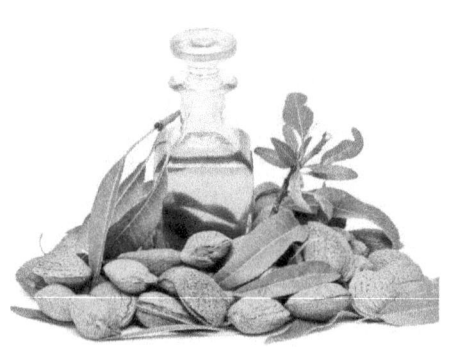

Almond oil is a rich source of vitamin E that not only enriches your health but also deeply nourishes your skin, giving it a youthful appearance. Try a daily massage with almond oil to treat dry and scaly skin on your feet. However, people who are allergic to nuts should avoid its use, as it may result in an allergic reaction.

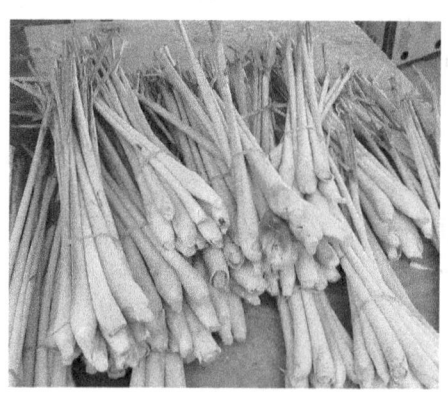

Lemongrass - This simple spice is extremely useful in relieving foot stress and soothing all kinds of muscle cramps and pain in your feet. It relaxes tired feet muscles and also deeply cleanses your skin. Use some lemongrass oil or raw paste in a tub of warm water as a foot bath to soothe your nerves and relax your feet.

Rosemary Oil - Rosemary is one of the most fragrant essential oils, and has powerful antifungal properties. In ancient times, rosemary oil was used as an effective stimulant of blood circulation and of mental concentration. Being an antibacterial, this oil helps cure strong bacterial/fungal infections and other conditions of the skin such as infected eczema, sores, yeast infections, calluses, and corns. A foot massage with this oil gives amazing relief. It can also be used in a tub of warm water with a few other medicinal essential oils.

Grape Seed Oil - This oil is mildly astringent in nature and is very useful in eliminating various fungal and bacterial infections of the skin, especially of the feet. The oil clears the blocked pores of your skin thoroughly and helps with the healing and repair of the skin layers. It also moisturizes the skin beautifully.

Garlic – A potent antibacterial and antifungal, garlic is one of the most powerful spices in your kitchen. It is a natural antifungal that rapidly reduces any kind of yeast infection. It is an effective remedy for athlete's foot. Apply raw garlic paste or oil on the affected part every day for a few days, and you will see the difference very quickly. Eating a few cloves of garlic every day boosts immunity, making you much less prone to yeast infection. You can even sprinkle garlic powder inside your socks and shoes for rapid action. The downside is its pungent odor; barring this, it is a highly recommended cure for any yeast infection.

Lavender Oil - Lavender oil has been of great importance to humankind for ages. The lavender plant is an extremely valuable medicinal plant that was discovered during the Roman era. Lavender oil is known to have great healing and antiseptic qualities. The oil is also known for its fragrant aroma. Lavender is used mainly for treating all kinds of skin conditions. It is also therapeutic in ailments like migraines, headaches, burns, stomach ailments, insect bites, muscle aches, and joint pains. It is especially powerful in athlete's foot. Lavender relieves stress and nervous strain and has a calming effect on the body. And besides,

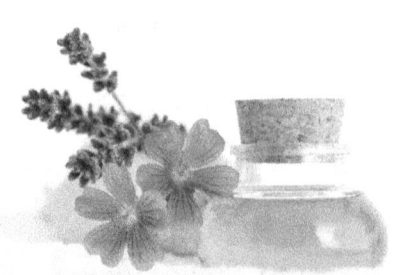 it gets the blood pumping! If your feet are stressed and weary, pamper yourself with a lavender foot soak. If you have athlete's foot, massage pure lavender oil on the affected part every day. It soothes the irritation and prevents the spread of infection to other parts of the body.

Cornstarch - Cornstarch is another wonderful kitchen ingredient that helps remove foot odor efficiently. It acts in the same capacity as baking soda and provides the same benefits. Sprinkle as much cornstarch powder as you need inside your smelly shoes to eliminate odor. The cornstarch powder absorbs excess moisture from your shoes and deodorizes them. You can also dust some powder inside your socks to control the accumulation of perspiration from your feet.

Jojoba Oil - This essential oil is known to have superb moisturizing properties. Jojoba oil is used in many beauty preparations because of its cleansing and conditioning qualities. Moreover, this oil is completely fragrance free. It naturally blends with your skin and deeply conditions it, making it supple and soft. It is a great cure for dry and cracked heels.

Tea Tree Oil – This is one of the most powerful herbal essential oils, with potent antifungal and antibacterial properties. It is widely used as an effective home remedy for a variety of fungal/yeast infections. It is also a very powerful immunity booster that is used to heal deep-seated infections. It completely relieves foot conditions like athlete's foot and eczema. Regular use of tea tree oil greatly benefits these foot conditions and prevents their recurrence.

Sea Salt* - This salt is rich in a variety of minerals, contains many marine extracts and has remarkable skin healing properties. Sea salt is an excellent exfoliating agent and can be used for home-based pedicure treatments. It helps gently loosen the hardened skin layers of your soles, making your feet smooth and soft. It additionally helps stimulate the circulation of blood in your feet to a great extent.

Oregano Oil - Oregano oil is a strong essential oil that is used for treating all kinds of yeast infections. Oregano is popularly used as a flavoring ingredient because of its spicy aroma and taste. However, it is a great immunity booster, too. Oregano oil can be used both topically and orally for curing yeast infections. The oil may be applied directly or after dilution with a little bland oil (such as olive oil) for sensitive skin. It can also be taken internally to strengthen your immunity. It has been known to completely cure yeast infections.

Yogurt - Yogurt is one of the most common of all these remedies, and yet it is one of the strongest fighters against all kinds of yeast and bacterial infections. Yogurt contains active Lactobacillus acidophilus bacteria that prevent the growth of bad yeasts of all kinds in the human body. It also kills yeasts that have infected the body. Yogurt has a marked cooling and soothing effect on the body. It can be applied externally on the affected part to reduce the irritation, itching, and stinging symptoms of yeast infections. If you have a yeast infection, be sure to include plenty of unsweetened yogurt in your diet.

Avocado Oil - Avocado is a rich source of vitamins A, D, and E and is known to treat dry skin conditions very effectively. Avocado oil has deep moisturizing effects on your skin, leaving it extremely soft and silky smooth. This contributes to its anti-aging properties too. It contains proteins, lecithin*, potassium, and unsaturated fatty acids* that add to the beauty and health of your skin. It can be used in a tub of warm water for a foot soak to treat cracked heels and soles, or for a foot massage. It can also be used for foot baths and home pedicures.

Shea Butter - This is a highly popular beauty ingredient best known for its remarkable moisturizing properties. Shea butter contains natural latex that is used in many moisturizing lotions and creams. Regularly applying lotions or creams based on shea butter is a very effective way to treat dry and cracked feet. It heals and deeply moisturizes dry skin, including heel cracks and fissures.

Peppermint Oil - This well-known essential oil is widely used to cure several ailments. Peppermint oil is known for its refreshing and cooling properties, which are useful in conditions like muscle aches, heel pains, foot pains, nausea symptoms, cough, cold, sinus, and headaches. The oil is generally applied topically on the affected area and has an amazing rejuvenating and healing effect.

Coconut Oil - Coconut oil is a very common household treatment for yeast infections. It has excellent antimicrobial properties. When this oil is applied on the infected region as many times as possible, the results will be visible in a few days. The oil has a pleasantly invigorating aroma. The flesh and water are both delicious and healthy. It has anti-aging properties and is an excellent skin moisturizer and conditioner. It can be combined with other essential oils to create a strong antifungal mix.

Cranberries - Cranberries have strong antibacterial and antifungal properties. Their tangy acidic content make them an ideal choice for treating every kind of fungi infection. Cranberry juice is usually recommended for treating yeast and bacterial infections. Make unsweetened cranberry juice a daily staple, and have plenty of it if you have a yeast infection. The acidic juice fights the fungus and flushes out the body system, preventing further fungal growth. The results will be obvious within days.

Vinegar - Vinegar is also an excellent antifungal. The most commonly used varieties for treating yeast infections are apple cider vinegar and white vinegar. Soaking your infected feet in a warm solution of either of these will quickly soothe skin irritations and itching. If you wish, you can soak a cotton ball in the diluted vinegar and apply it on the affected area several times a day.

Olive Leaf - Olive leaf extract is a popular and effective treatment for fighting a yeast infection. It has antiviral, anti-inflammatory, and antioxidant properties. It effectively eliminates the bad fungi in your body and restores the good bacteria. Olive leaf extract can be easily made at home. Chopped fresh olive leaves are put into a glass container and vodka is added to extract the oil. Close the mixture tightly and store the jar in a cool, dark place for a

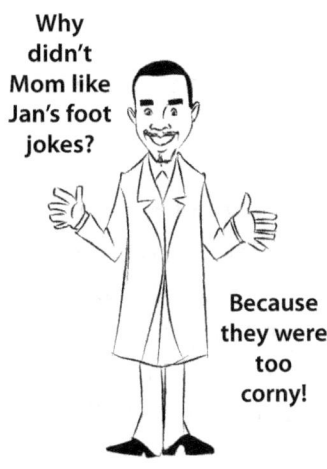

Why didn't Mom like Jan's foot jokes?

Because they were too corny!

month. Then, strain the leaves out. The liquid can be decanted*
into a fresh glass container and stored. If this extract is applied
on the infected part every day, the results will be visible within
a few weeks.

Calendula - Calendula is another herbal remedy for fighting fungal infections. Calendula is a medicinal plant with effective anti-inflammatory and antibacterial properties. To obtain
best results, it should be applied in its pure raw form. Calendula
petals are made into a paste and applied to the affected area.
This soothes the itching and burning sensations. It can also be
taken internally as calendula tea. This will boost your immune
response and enable faster healing. Calendula oil, ointment, or
lotions are all available for use, and you can pick and choose
among these.

Baking Soda - Baking soda is an old remedy for foot odor,
which affects a large chunk of the population. It can be dusted
inside your shoes and left overnight. It will absorb moisture and
eliminate the foul smell from your shoes. If you want to add
some fragrance to your shoes, you can mix it with some sweet-
smelling herbs like sage or lavender. These herbs will contribute their efficacious antifungal properties to protect you from all
kinds of yeast and other fungal infections.

Ginger - Another essential kitchen ingredient is ginger. Antibacterial and antiseptic, ginger helps fight fungal infections and
soothe foot pain and swelling. It is a very good natural remedy
for arthritis and joint pain. Grate a generous quantity of ginger
and boil it in water to extract the essence. This solution can be
used as a foot dip to soothe your aching feet and stimulate circulation as well as to restore warmth to cold feet. Another way
to use it is by tying up a quantity of mashed ginger in a soft

cotton cloth, which is then dipped into a bowl of hot water. Rub this all over your feet just before you go to bed and let it soak in overnight.

Radish - Radish is an excellent deodorizer in your kitchen. To remove foot odor, extract as much radish juice as you need. You can store it in a spray bottle. Add a little glycerin to preserve it. This can be sprayed onto your feet after washing them thoroughly.

Black Tea - Black tea is a very popular cure for feet perspiration. Black tea contains tannic acid, with strong astringent properties that inhibit foot sweating. It is prepared as a foot soak by dipping around 6 tea bags in a tub of hot water. After it has cooled for a few minutes, add ice cubes to it. Let your feet soak in this cold solution for about half an hour. Repeat this procedure daily, especially during the summertime. It provides great comfort and coolness to your feet.

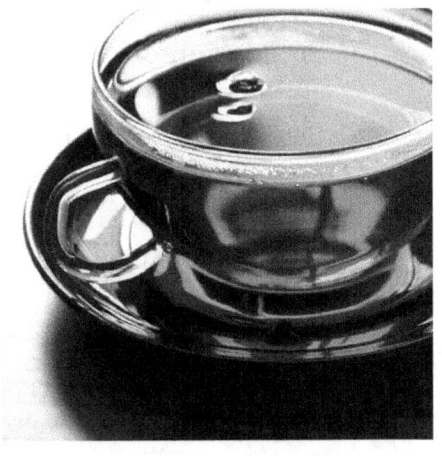

Water - An alternate hot and cold water bath is one of the most effective ways to reduce stress, pain, and sweaty feet conditions. A little lemon juice added to the water adds an astringent property, helping to clean the pores of your skin thoroughly. Fill two tubs, one with hot water and the other with icy-cold water. Add the juice of one whole lemon to each tub. Find a comfortable seat. Dip your feet first in the hot water and then in the cold, until your feet are relaxed and pain-free. Take breaks for a minute or two in between. Once you are comfortable, finish off with a final hot water dip. Dry your feet gently, but thoroughly, with a clean towel. Dust them with herbal powder. This treatment really works for foot stress, especially during the hot summer months.

Chaparral - Chaparral is a desert plant with very powerful antifungal properties. The leaves of this plant can cure even the severest forms of fungal infections. A raw paste made from crushed chaparral leaves is applied directly on fungal/bacterial infections on the skin. Fungal infections like athlete's foot, and skin conditions like eczema, itching, and other skin irritations are effectively treated with chaparral. Chaparral can also be used for treating fungal infections in other parts of the body like the scalp or the fingernails.

Black Walnut - Black Walnut is another useful treatment for fungal infections of the feet. Its beneficial properties include antifungal, antibacterial, anti-inflammatory, and antiseptic qualities. It can be applied topically on the affected part, and both soothes and heals the skin.

Thyme - Thyme is a popular herb from your kitchen that fights fungal infections very well. Thyme is not only treasured in traditional cuisine but also used as a very important ingredient in herbal medicinal preparations. It has strong antiseptic properties and treats a variety of fungal infections.

Neem - Neem is a common yet extremely potent antifungal herb. Neem is found mainly in tropical countries and is widely used for its amazing antiseptic, antifungal, and antibacterial properties. It is very versatile and is used in many herbal preparations. Every part of the neem tree - including the leaves, stems, roots, and flowers - are used in a variety of ways. Neem has a very bitter taste. A paste of raw neem leaves can be applied topically to reduce fungal infections. Neem juice is great to detoxify your system. Neem application gives speedy healing results for fungal infections, eczema, and inflammations of the skin.

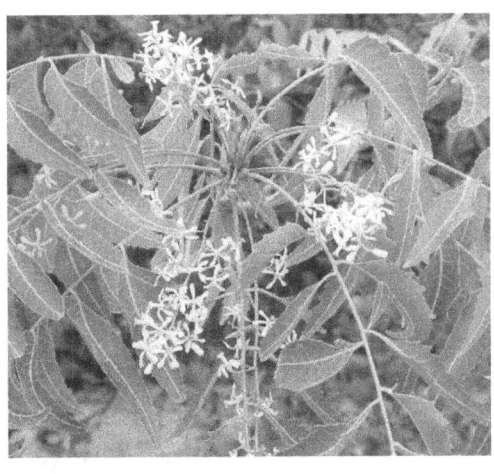

Cayenne Pepper - Cayenne pepper is a spicy ingredient in your kitchen that helps treat cold feet symptoms effectively. When applied topically on your feet, it stimulates heat production and blood circulation. If you suffer from cold feet, just dust some cayenne pepper powder inside your socks before you wear them; your feet will instantly warm up. But remember to change your socks daily, as using the pepper might stain them. Wash your hands thoroughly, as it will burn if the powder comes into contact with your eyes.

Chamomile Oil - Chamomile is a very potent painkiller with remarkable anti-inflammatory properties. It is markedly useful for treating foot problems like blisters, bunions, inflammation, burns, boils, allergies, itching, and common foot wounds. Chamomile is a very mild herb that not only soothes skin discomfort and pain but also helps in regeneration of tissues, thus aiding the process of healing. It is also a good antibiotic, antiseptic, antibacterial, and antidepressant. Chamomile oil also moisturizes dry skin well.

Eucalyptus - Eucalyptus is an herb with very strong antibacterial actions. It is widely used for treating various fungal and bacterial infections. The oil has a penetrating mint-like aroma and is used for its warming effect on the skin. It also helps relieve muscle pain, sores, arthritis, rheumatic pain, foot swelling, and sprains. Spraying your bathroom and kitchen floor with eucalyptus oil disinfects these areas naturally. It is also extremely useful in relieving congestion of the sinuses, and in coughs and colds. It is not advised for those who have high blood pressure or epilepsy, because of its strong stimulant action.

Cypress - Cypress is a useful essential oil that is derived from the cypress plant, found mainly in the Mediterranean regions. The oil has a woodsy and musky fragrance. Its uses lie in its antiseptic, astringent, antispasmodic, and deodorant properties. It is used to treat excessive foot perspiration, foot odor, and varicose* veins. It soothes the skin and helps in relieving stress and skin irritations. It is also highly therapeutic for arthritis and rheumatic pain. Put a few drops of this oil in your footbath before you soak your feet. You can even use it in your bath to relax your overstrung nerves.

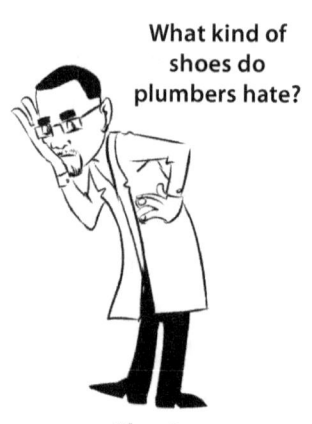

What kind of shoes do plumbers hate?

Clogs!

Clary Sage - Clary sage essential oil is derived from the Salvia sclarea plant. Though the plant is a rare one, its oil has many medicinal properties. Clary sage oil is pale yellow with a very sweet and nutty aroma. This oil is very therapeutic because of its properties as an antiseptic, deodorant, astringent, antibacterial, and nerve tonic*. It soothes the nerves of the legs and feet, relieves muscle pain and cramps, and effectively treats skin inflammation and blisters. Use a few drops of this oil in your footbath or massage it directly on your feet to feel the difference.

Geranium - Geranium oil is a widely used herbal remedy for foot infections, whether bacterial or fungal. It is derived from the Pelargonium odoratissimum plant. There are more than seven hundred varieties of this plant, but only ten are used for medicinal purposes. The oil has a very strong and fresh aroma that slightly resembles mint. It is widely used in aromatherapy, being an active antiseptic, deodorant, anti-inflammatory, astringent, and tonic. It is a powerful stimulator of blood circulation in your feet. Massaging your feet with this oil will help relieve conditions like sore heels, foot swelling, bunions, blisters, edema, inflammation, burns, and cuts. It is also a very good insect repellent.

Cinnamon - Cinnamon oil is a popular essential oil that has been used since ancient times in Egypt, India, Ceylon, and Indonesia. This exotic oil has great healing properties that include antiseptic, antibiotic, astringent, and deodorizing effects. Cinnamon is used in a wide variety of herbal preparations. It is also widely used in aromatherapy because of its strong, musky, and spicy fragrance that rejuvenates the mind and body, and relieves exhaustion and stress. It is very helpful in relieving arthritis and rheumatic disorders of the feet. It is also used in foot massage therapy to stimulate blood circulation. It is useful in all kinds of muscular foot pains and cramps. It can also be used with other essential oils for therapeutic purposes. Since cinnamon oil is strong and spicy, it must be diluted before use to avoid skin irritations.

Juniper Berry - Juniper oil is used for treating contagious feet conditions like eczema, athlete's foot, inflammation, and other fungal infections. Juniper is extracted from Juniperus communis, the common juniper plant. The oil is an astringent, antifungal, antiseptic, anti-rheumatic, and tonic. Juniper oil can be used in footbaths for treating arthritis and eczema. It also calms and mollifies the skin. Seeping deep into the pores of your skin, it releases muscular stress and tension and enhances blood circulation. It also relieves edema by reducing fluid retention in your feet.

Lemon Oil - Lemon oil is one of the most common and widely used essential oils. It is extracted from the Citrus limonum plant and is also popularly known as Cedro oil. Lemon has a very clean, refreshing, and fresh fragrance. The therapeutic properties of lemon oil are due to its antimicrobial, antiseptic,

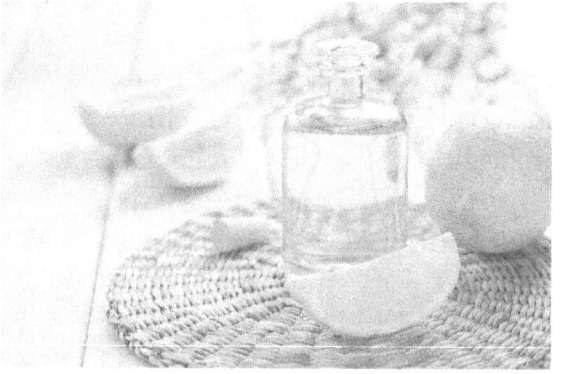 disinfectant, stimulant, and tonic functions. Lemon oil is of great use in relieving foot problems like arthritis, gout, rheumatic pains, boils, blisters, swelling, and fungal infections. It is a great stimulant to the circulation of blood in the feet. A good warm footbath with a few drops of lemon essential oil aids in releasing stress from your feet, effectively soothing and cleaning them. It additionally helps fight foot odor and heals insect bites. Lemon oil can also be used to treat minor cuts and injuries in your foot.

Benzoin Oil - Benzoin oil is good for relieving itchiness, redness, swelling, dryness, and other irritations of the skin. This essential oil is extracted from the resin of the Styrax benzoin tree, which is a native of the Asian islands of Java, Sumatra, and Thailand. It is also popularly known as Gum Benzoin or Frankincense of Java. The oil has a very warm, woody vanilla-like aroma and is deep golden-brown in color. Benzoin oil is used as an astringent, antiseptic, anti-inflammatory, and anti-rheumatic. Benzoin oil is remarkably useful in foot conditions like arthritis, rheumatism, eczema, athlete's foot, heel pain, and foot odor. It stimulates the nervous system and boosts the circulation of blood in the body. It soothes foot symptoms like pain and swelling, itching, redness, and inflammation. It is also a great skin conditioner and helps heal the dry and cracked soles of your feet, making the dry skin supple and soft. The warming effect of benzoin oil is very useful for treating arthritic and rheumatic pains in the feet. It also effectively activates the stiff muscles resulting from neuropathy, as well as the nerves themselves. Benzoin oil is of special benefit to diabetic patients, as it helps control blood sugar levels. It also heals common wounds and cuts on the feet.

Sandalwood - Sandalwood oil is one of the most exotic essential oils. Sandalwood oil is extracted from the sandalwood tree that is found mainly in the Indian sub-continent. Sandalwood oil has been used in ancient Indian Ayurvedic medicine for its great healing and therapeutic properties. The oil has an exotic and subtle woody aroma that is very soothing. The oil itself has antiseptic, antibacterial, astringent, and deodorizing properties. The healing and soothing properties of this oil helps relieve feet conditions like eczema, dryness, inflammation, itching, and stress. The oil also has marvelous anti-aging properties that not only cleanse the skin on your feet but also give it a youthful glow. The strong essence of sandalwood is extremely beneficial in banishing foot odor. Massaging this oil into your feet every day will help relieve nervous strain and aches in your feet. The oil also helps repair and diminish ugly scars caused by blisters and eczema* infections on your feet.

Neroli - Neroli essential oil, popularly known as orange blossom oil, is derived from the orange flower tree. Neroli oil is one of the most fragrant essential oils, next only to lavender, in addition to its therapeutic properties. Its aroma is both exquisitely sweet and rejuvenating. It is widely used in aromatherapy to soothe and calm the body and mind. It also has antiseptic, antibacterial, deodorant, and anti-stress properties. Neroli oil helps remove dry eczema scars and other types of foot scars very effectively. Its marvelous skin-regenerating properties give a glow to the skin. It is a great treatment for foot odor. Just a few drops of Neroli oil in your warm water footbath will deodorize your feet as well as soothe and refresh your skin.

Basil - Basil is a very useful herbal plant. It originated mainly in India and is still regarded as a very sacred plant in Hindu tradition. The essential oil from basil is extracted from Common, or Sweet Basil, which grows mostly in tropical climatic regions.

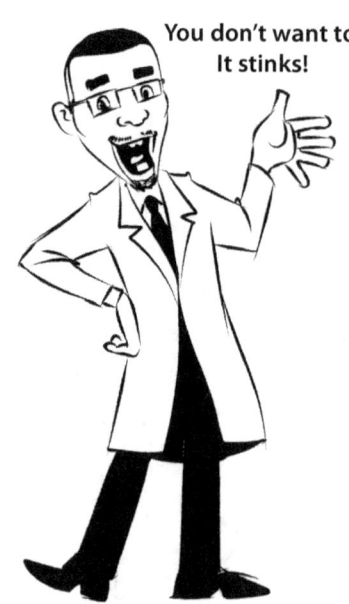

Did you hear the joke about the gym socks?

You don't want to. It stinks!

The oil is popularly used in aromatherapy to calm the nerves and treat migraines, headaches, and sinus or bronchial problems. Basil oil is pale green with a very refreshing, sweet pepper-like aroma. It has antibacterial, antiseptic, deodorizing, analgesic, stimulant, and insect repellent properties. Basil oil is highly effective in the treatment of fungal infections like eczema, athlete's foot, toenail fungus, inflammation, redness, itching, burning, gout, and arthritis. Basil can also be taken internally to reduce the uric acid levels in the body and thus relieve gout pain. It can relieve arthritic pains and stimulate blood circulation. It reduces any type of external foot infection, whether fungal or resulting from insect bites.

Ylang-Ylang - Ylang-Ylang oil is a well-known essential oil that is famous for its wonderful sweet aroma and widely used in aromatherapy. It is mainly found in the Asiatic islands of Java, Sumatra, and Thailand. The therapeutic properties of this oil are antiseptic, antifungal, deodorant, and stimulant. Ylang-Ylang oil is immensely beneficial in curing foot pain, stressed feet, and dry, flaky skin. Soak your feet in warm water with a few drops of Ylang-Ylang oil to experience the deep calming effect on your feet. This oil also nourishes very dry skin on your feet, perfectly balancing the skin's pH level to make it supple and smooth again. It also banishes foot odor effectively.

Bergamot - Bergamot oil is a popular aromatherapy oil used to relieve stress. It is used in spas to treat skin allergies and rashes effectively. Bergamot is mainly found in regions of Southeast Asia and in some parts of Europe. The greenish-yellow oil has an incredible warm and fruity citrus aroma. The therapeutic properties of this oil are antiseptic, antibiotic, anti-bacterial, deodorant, and analgesic*. It helps with foot conditions like eczema, rashes and allergic reactions on the feet. Its antiseptic property helps clean cuts and wounds of all kinds. It should be diluted before use on sensitive skin, as it may otherwise be irritating.

Frankincense - Frankincense oil is an exotic essential oil used in aromatherapy to calm the mind and body. Its wonderful healing properties revive the body incredibly. The oil is extracted from the resin of the Boswellia carteri tree, found mainly in the Middle East. The yellowish-green oil has a spicy, camphoric aroma with a woody essence. The healing properties of this oil are anti-rheumatic, analgesic, antiseptic, astringent*, and stimulant. It is highly beneficial in the treatment of rheumatism because of the way it relieves muscular aches and pains. Frankincense oil can also be used for treating arthritis and all other kinds of foot pain, sores, itching, inflammation, blisters, and burns. The warming effect of the oil is a great stimulant and improves blood circulation in your feet. It is also endowed with special anti-aging and deep conditioning properties that help restore your skin's softness and suppleness. Frankincense oil can be used in diluted and undiluted form in foot baths and foot massages as well as in creams or ointments.

Chapter 5

Foot Care In Summer And Winter

F oot care should be an essential part of your daily routine. When seasons change, it becomes even more important. Your feet need special care during summer and winter. This will help you avoid many foot problems that crop up during these times. Here are some indispensable tips on foot care that will help you take much better care of your feet during the summer and winter.

Summer Foot Care Tips

Summer is a time for outdoor activities and adventure-filled vacations. It is at this time of the year that your feet are most exposed to the environment. Consequently, your feet are especially prone to developing many problems at this time, whether by catching an infection or just an ordinary skin issue. Basic precautions are essential to avoid much pain and discomfort. Listed below are some common summer foot problems, along with ways to prevent them.

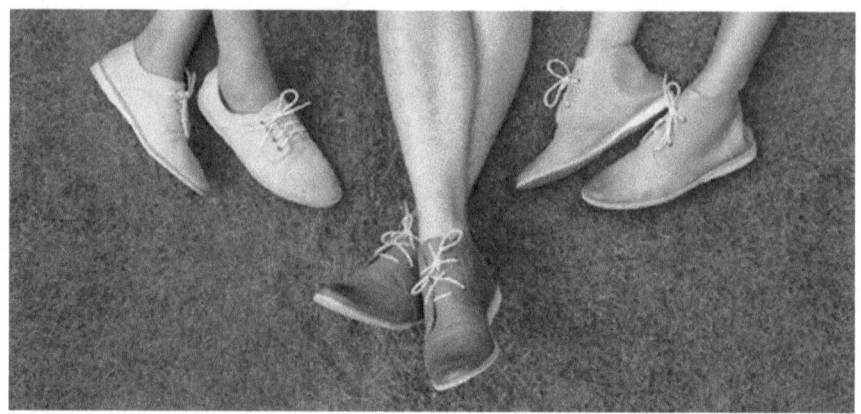

Wear Comfortable and Flexible Footwear to Avoid Blisters - Blisters are the most common foot problem occurring during the summer months. They usually occur because of the way socks and shoes keep rubbing against the surface of the skin. Blisters are mainly seen with new or ill-fitting shoes. Shoes that are too tight or narrow cause constant friction against your skin when you walk. The problem is aggravated by the scorching summer heat and perspiration. The skin responds to repetitive injury by the formation of painful blisters. This can be avoided by wearing comfortable and flexible footwear that allows your feet to breathe. It is also important to alternate between shoes, sandals, and flip-flops to keep your feet clean and dry. This helps prevent blisters from forming.

Wear Flip-Flops or Sandals in Public Pools and Showers - Public shower areas and wet swimming pool floors are breeding places for fungi, which can cause foot infections. Athlete's foot, fungal toenail, plantar warts, and so on are all common fungal infections that are contracted from places like these. Therefore, make sure you always wear sandals and flip-flops in these places to protect your feet. Never walk barefoot in these areas to avoid exposing your feet to such infections. Use waterproof footwear if you have an open wound in either of your feet, or any other foot problems that can expose your feet to such risks.

Take Regular Footbaths and Get Pedicures – Taking time to have regular foot baths and pedicures in the summer helps prevent a lot of foot problems. A pedicure helps exfoliate the dead skin and cleanse your feet. Gentle scraping and scrubbing are the two important pedicure procedures that keep the skin of your feet healthy and improve the circulation of blood in your feet. A pedicure also includes a foot massage, which leads to intense relaxation and stimulates blood flow.

Taking foot baths will release your feet from the day's exhaustion and stress. After a tiring day, soaking your feet in good warm water with a few drops of essential oil can work absolute magic, driving away every trace of stress and fatigue from your feet. If you have foot pain, try taking alternate hot water and cold water baths to relieve the pain.

Trim your Toenails - During the summer it is very important to trim and cut your toenails short. Since your feet are always in contact with the ground, they accumulate a lot of dirt and germs. Long nails increase the risk of contracting fungal infections like toenail fungus and foot odor. On the other hand, keeping your nails short and clean is the safest way to avoid such infections. You should also wash your feet regularly with mild antibacterial soaps and dust them with antifungal herbal powders to keep fungal infections at bay.

Keep Your Feet Dry - Perspiration is an inevitable part of the hot and humid summer months. If your feet perspire a lot in the summer, try to keep your feet as dry as possible to avoid foot odors and discourage fungal growth on your feet. Regularly soak your feet in warm water containing Epsom salts or kosher salt since these salts are endowed with special properties to limit the amount of perspiration. Afterwards, dry your feet thoroughly with a towel and then dust some fragrant talcum powder on your feet. When you go outdoors, dust some cornstarch powder inside your socks. Its high absorbency will help keep perspiration from accumulating inside your shoes.

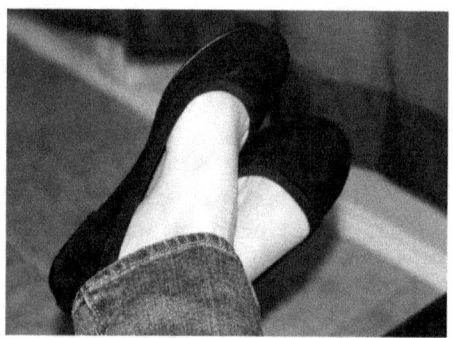

Wear Comfortable and Well-Fitting Shoes - Wear shoes that keep your feet dry and comfortable during the summer. Open top shoes like sandals, floaters, flip-flops, and light canvas shoes are the best footwear during this season. Summer activities like cycling, walking, jogging, and afternoon beach walks can be enjoyable with the right kind of footwear.

Use a Good Sunscreen - Since your feet are the most exposed parts of your body, they are prone to tanning. The use of a good tanning lotion or a high-quality sunscreen will protect the skin texture of your feet. Regular use of sunscreen will make sure you don't get unwanted spots, dark patches, and tanning over your feet. If you can, wear light and soft seamless socks outdoors to protect your feet from the direct UV rays of the sun.

Winter Foot Care Tips

Common foot problems associated with the winter season are stiffness, aching joints, leg cramps, cracked heels and fissures, and dry skin. It is important to protect your feet from the cold as much as you can to help maintain your natural body heat. Feet are highly susceptible to winter damage. Therefore, it is essential to keep them covered and warm at all times. If you suffer from cold feet or arthritic pains, it is even more important to keep your feet warm. Since warmth enhances blood circulation, problems like muscle cramps and stiffness of joints and tendons are less likely to occur if your legs and feet are covered and protected.

Wear Socks and Shoes All the Time - Wearing socks and shoes help your feet remain warm and comfortable. It also protects your feet from frostbite and numbness. Make sure that you wear socks at bedtime, too, to keep your feet warm all through the night. If the weather is very chilly, wear thick socks. Socks should be made from natural fabrics like cotton and wool. Avoid wearing tight socks, as this will hamper the blood circulation to your feet and cause them to feel cold. They can induce leg cramps as well. Loose, comfortable, seamless socks are ideal.

Wash Your Feet Daily - Keeping your feet clean is also very important in the winter. Washing your feet at least once a day with lukewarm water will keep them healthy and hygienic.

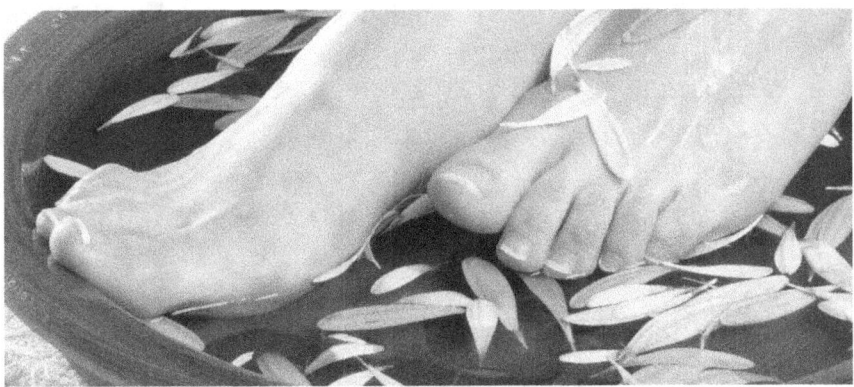

However, do not use very hot water, as this may strip natural oils from your skin and leave it dry. After washing your feet, dry them gently, but thoroughly, and then apply a good moisturizer on both sides of your feet (but not between your toes) to keep your skin hydrated.

Moisturize Your Feet Daily - Dry feet are common in winter. Your feet can appear rough, scaly, and cracked. Sometimes they are also painful or itchy. The best way to avoid this is a daily moisturizing ritual using a good foot lotion or cream that will help maintain the pH balance of your skin. Washing your feet with soap, especially during winter, leaves the skin dry; applying a good lotion or cream helps lock in the natural moisture and keeps the skin smooth and supple. The areas most likely to show the effects of dryness are the heels and soles. Cracks and fissures often develop in these areas if the skin dries out for a long time. The earlier a crack is attended to, the better, since delayed treatment allows them to deepen and extend into the underlying tissues as well. This can be an invitation to serious foot infections. All this can be easily avoided by the regular use of a good moisturizing agent.

What kind of shoes do lazy people wear? Loafers.

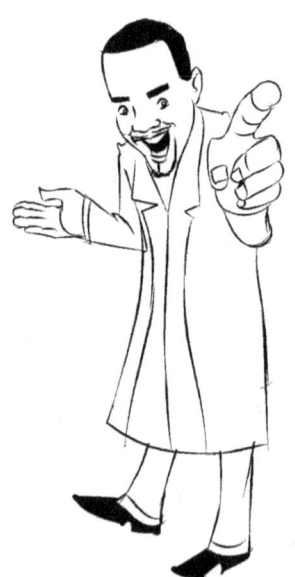

Warm Ups - Exercising your foot muscles is an essential part of foot care, especially during the winter months. This keeps your muscles and tendons from stiffening up with the cold. Exercise warms up the feet, makes the muscles and tendons strong and flexible, and increases the circulation of blood. These beneficial changes in turn protect your feet from sudden injury during rapid movement. Serious foot conditions like diabetic foot or arthritis demand that you make exercise an integral part of your daily winter routine to avoid joint stiffness and loss of foot sensation.

Use a Foot Scrub - Use a pumice stone or a foot scrub to gently peel off the dead layers of your skin. Since cracks are common in winter, it is important to remove the accumulated layers of dead skin at regular intervals to avoid fungal infection of the non-viable tissue. Remember to be gentle. Hard scrubbing may peel off living skin and expose the tissue to injury and infection. Once you have exfoliated your feet, apply a good moisturizer that will restore the vital and natural oils of your skin. Wear socks and sandals after every scrubbing session to protect your feet from dirt and cold.

Wear Thick Footwear - Winter is the time when you can show off those burnished, long leather boots. Wearing thicker shoes helps protect your feet from the biting cold. A thicker pair of warm socks will give you more insulation and protect your feet from the chilly weather by keeping away frostbite, cold sores, and stiffness of the legs.

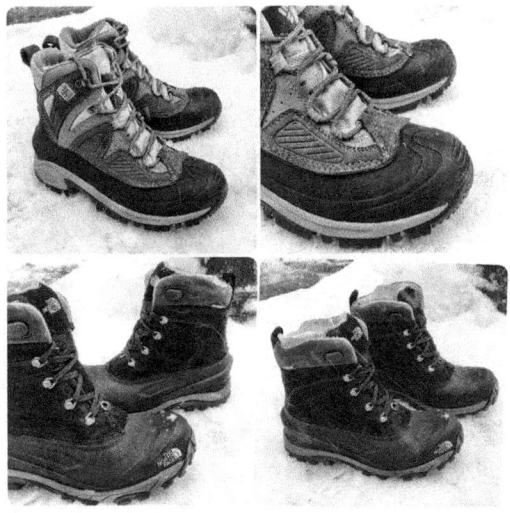

Chapter 6

Reflexology

F oot reflexology has been used for centuries, the earliest findings dating from Egypt in 2300 B.C.

Reflexology is a gentle therapy used to help restore and maintain your body's natural equilibrium.

Reflexology isn't capable of curing any serious or life-threatening medical disorder and does not claim to cure, diagnose or prescribe; however as an alternative healing method, it is extremely popular with people from all walks of life.

Who Can Benefit from Reflexology?

Reflexology is suitable for all.

Many people use reflexology as a means of relaxing the mind and body and it has been shown to be an effective tool for, stress related conditions, sleep disorders, back pain, migraine, sleep disorders, digestive disorders, hormonal imbalances and arthritis

With stress being so prevalent in our society today, this gentle, soothing therapy provides a method of stress release that can help on a physical, mental and emotional level.

How Does Reflexology Work?

By stimulating and applying pressure to the feet or hands, reflexology increases circulation and can promote specific bodily and muscular functions.

The hands and feet are more sensitive than most people realize. A professionally trained reflexologist can detect subtle changes in specific points on the feet, and by working on these points may affect the corresponding organ or system of the body.

Studies have shown reflexology to make improvements in physical and emotional movements, increase self esteem and confidence and improve the ability to stay motivated and improve concentration. What Happens During a Reflexology Session?

According to Chinese medicine, the soles of the feet hold the sensory nerves of the internal organs that are spread through the body.

During a reflexology session, the therapist applies manual pressure to the feet, working on specific points that connect with different zones in your body.

Pressure is then applied to particular areas of the soles of the feet.

FOOT REFLEXOLOGY CHART

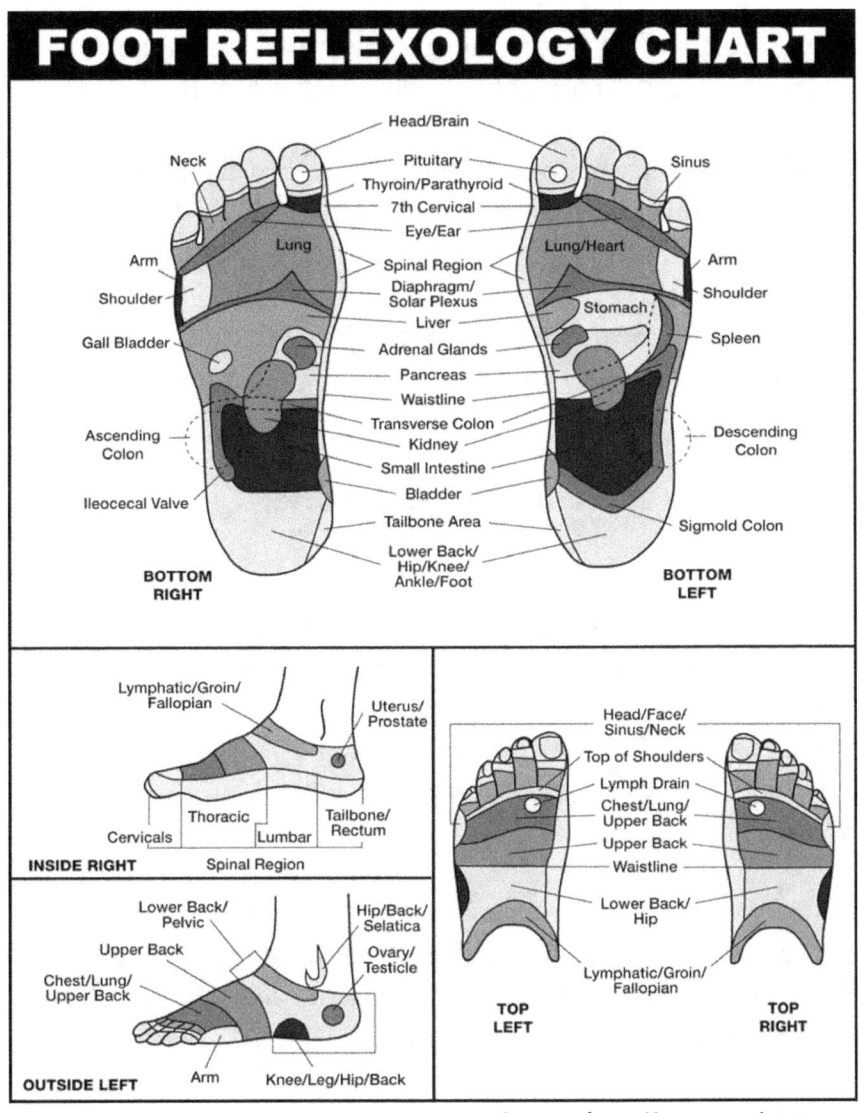

Source: http://www.puristat.com

Deposits and imbalances are sought out and released in order to remove blockages and restore the flow of blood and energy.

Reflexology uses hands, fingers, a wooden stick, cream, and oils to stimulate a reflex action in another part of the body.

When properly practiced, reflexology gives a feeling of well-being and relaxation as it stimulates the body to help heal itself.

You should wear loose comfortable clothes that are unrestricting as only your shoes and socks will be removed.

Reflexology - is it safe for everyone?

If you have a heart condition, diabetes, epilepsy, high blood pressure or kidney problems, you should consult your healthcare provider before embarking on a course of reflexology.

Pregnant or menstruating women and people who are bleeding either internally or externally should not receive reflexology

Reflexology massage can be given every day but only for a duration of 45 minutes. You should begin to experience a positive difference after one or two treatments. Most people experience a feeling of relaxation and wellbeing.

Occasionally people report feelings of nausea, tearfulness or feeling lethargic after a reflexology session. Therapists say this is part of the healing process.

It is important that you report any of these feelings to your reflexology therapist so that he or she can adopt your treatment plan accordingly.

Reflexology should be avoided for at least one hour after meals. As with most massage therapies you should drink plenty of water after treatment.

Many people use reflexology as a means of relaxing the mind and body and it has grown in popularity in recent years as way of relaxing and de-stressing from the pressures we all face on a day to day basis.

Reflexology - Finding a Therapist

To get the best from a reflexology session you should seek out a suitably trained therapist. Most Spas, salons and health clubs now offer massage treatments and some therapist will carry out a reflexology treatment in the comfort of your own home.

- www.skin-care-recipes-and-remedies.com

Chapter 7

Daily Essential Foot Care Tips

n this chapter, I want to pass on some valuable guidelines for daily foot care. I will also provide a few recipes for natural homemade foot pack recipes. But first, the tips for daily basic foot care.

Washing – Washing your feet daily with mild soap and water is a vital step towards maintaining healthy and disease-free feet. A daily cleansing routine helps wash away the accumulated dirt and microbes on your feet. The warm water helps open up the blocked pores on the surface of your skin and ensures a thorough cleansing.

Examine Your Feet – It is very important to examine your feet regularly for any visible abnormality. If your nail color changes from white to yellow, purple, or black it might indicate the fungal growth. Check your heels and toes for any cracks or cuts. A regular evaluation of your feet will help you detect such anomalies early so they can be promptly treated.

Trim Toenails – Trimming your toenails is a healthy habit. Long toenails not only look unkempt but also gather a lot of dirt and germs, making your feet smelly and unsightly, as well as susceptible to foot diseases like toenail fungus, athlete's foot, infected eczema, and so on.

Wear Good-Fitting Shoes – Wear shoes that are comfortable and provide good support to your feet. Do not compromise the health of your feet for the sake of fashion or style. Women especially should avoid wearing very high heels, which can cause serious foot impairment and eventually restrict foot mobility.

Throw Out Old Pairs – Do not wear worn out and broken down shoes or sneakers. They offer no support, and this will damage the feet. Also, they will harbor bacteria and fungus; toss them and buy a new well-fitting pair of shoes or sneakers.

Change Daily – Do not wear the same pair of shoes every day, as this increases the probability of fungal infection. Foot odor also arises from repeatedly wearing the same footwear all the time. Alternate between two or more pairs of shoes so that one pair can be dried in the sun and cleaned well before it needs to be used again. Sun exposure will deodorize your shoes and will help reduce microbes.

Apply Sunscreen - Your feet are prone to tanning just like the rest of your body. Therefore, use a good sunscreen on your feet if you wear sandals or flip-flops outdoors.

Wear Good Quality Fabrics – Use socks made from natural fabrics like cotton and wool. These allow your feet to breathe and are gentle on your skin. Women should avoid wearing tight nylon hose and stockings to keep from hampering blood circulation in the legs and feet.

Who always goes to bed with his shoes on?

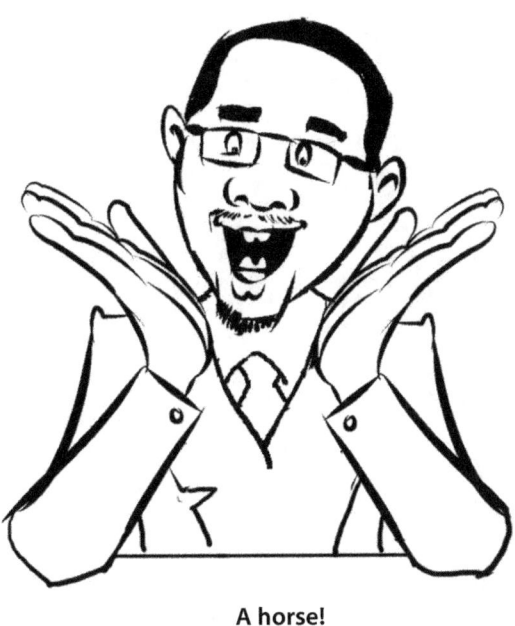

A horse!

Chapter 8

Natural Homemade Foot Care Recipes

1. Homemade Feet Toner & Cleanser

Ingredients: The juice of two big lemons, warm water, tissue paper.

Method: In a tumbler, mix equal quantities of lemon juice and warm water. Dip the tissues one by one into the solution and place them on your feet for a few minutes. Once the skin has had time to soak in the juice, remove the tissues gently, wiping off the skin as you do so.

Benefits: Lemon is a superb cleansing agent. The astringent properties of lemon act as a toner, helping to open up the clogged pores of your feet. The antiseptic property of the lemon not only deactivates fungal growth on your feet but also helps remove foot odor.

2. Homemade Foot Exfoliating Pack

Ingredients: 10 strawberries, 2 tablespoons lavender oil/peppermint oil, 1 teaspoon kosher salt, and ½ teaspoon crushed apricots.

Method: Blend all the ingredients in a mixer to form a thick paste. Pour it into a bowl and gently apply the paste with a circular rubbing motion all over your feet.

Benefits: This is an excellent scrub for treating dry skin conditions, cracks, and roughness of the feet.

3. Homemade Foot Lotion

Ingredients: 1 tablespoon almond oil, 1 tablespoon coconut oil, and a few drops of an essential oil of your choice (such as lavender or eucalyptus).

Method: Mix all the ingredients together in a dark bottle and shake it well until the oils are blended. Use this oil-based lotion on your feet every day, preferably after a foot bath, although it can be done at any time. Store the bottle in a cool, dark place.

Benefits: Coconut oil has great anti-aging properties, and almond oil is rich in vitamin E to help moisturize your feet and give them a youthful glow.

4. Homemade Foot Spa

Ingredients: The juice of two big lemons, 2 tablespoons coconut oil, half cup milk, half teaspoon cinnamon powder, and warm water.

Method: Mix all the ingredients with warm water in a foot basin. Give your feet a good soak in the aromatic solution for at least 20 minutes. Afterwards, wash your feet with soap and water. Pat them dry with a towel and apply a good moisturizer. Put on your socks immediately after the spa bath to preserve its effect.

Benefits: Coconut oil and milk helps make the texture of your feet feel soft and silky. You could make a foot spa part of your weekly routine.

5. My Special Foot Mask

Ingredients: Fresh avocado, massage oil, and honey.

Method: Mix ingredients together in a bowl, rub into both feet, allowing the mixture to stay on them for 10-15 minutes. Then use a foot basin to rinse.

Benefits: The natural oils in avocado penetrate deep into the skin, helping to soften and hydrate dry and flaky patches. With their healthy fats and phytonutrients, avocados offer remarkable benefits to human skin. Honey is a natural antioxidant, which proves beneficial when taken internally, but also provides protective benefits when used topically on the skin.

These simple tips and recipes show that putting a little care and time into foot care will help you achieve a beautiful and highly functional pair of feet. The home remedies mentioned here are very simple to follow, and the natural ingredients used are easily available in your kitchen. I hope these guidelines will help you save a lot of money on those visits to expensive salons for spas and pedicures.

The following spectacular foot care recipes are from www.skin-care-recipes-and-remedies.com

BROWN SUGAR FOOT SCRUB

Same as in the brown sugar body scrub, brown sugar helps slough off the dead skin cells.

Ingredients
- 2 tablespoons brown sugar
- 2 tablespoons ground oats
- 2 tablespoons aloe vera gel
- 1 tablespoon honey
- 1 teaspoon freshly squeezed lemon juice
- 1 teaspoon almond oil (in case you don't have almond oil, use olive oil, it is a great substitute).

Preparation
- ☛ Before you start preparing this scrub, grind the oatmeal using a coffee

grinder or food processor. It has to be of sandy consistency, flaky and light otherwise it will scratch the skin.

☞ Mix all the ingredients in a large bowl. Mix until it resembles a paste

☞ Use circular motion and massage gently.

☞ Rinse off with warm water.

SALT SCRUB

Ingredients
1 cup of sea salt or Epsom salt
1/2 cup of cold water
2 drops of lavender essential oil

Preparation
☞ Start off by gradually adding water to salt and lavender oil

☞ As you are adding it, you want to make sure the mix starts looking like a paste. It has to be not too liquid and not too solid, it should be like soft though otherwise it will run between your fingers

☞ Rub your feet and soles in circular motion

☞ Rinse off with warm water

The following two recipes are courtesy of Spaindex.com, the rest are from www.skin-care-recipes-and-remedies.com

HOMEMADE STRAWBERRY SCRUB

Ingredients
  8-10 strawberries
  2 tablespoons Apricot oil (you may
    substitute with olive oil
  1 teaspoon of coarse salt, such as
    Kosher salt, or Sea Salt

Preparation
  ☛ Mix all ingredients into a paste,
    massage into feet, rinse and pat dry

Note
This foot scrub is a great introduction
to application of homemade foot cream or
a store bought one for that purpose. Here
is a recipe to a wonderful overnight foot
masque.

OVERNIGHT FOOT MASQUE

Ingredients
  1/4 cup almonds
  1/4 dry oatmeal
  3 tablespoons food grade cocoa butter
  2 tablespoons honey

Preparation
  ☛ Process almonds in a blender or coffee
    grinder until finely ground
  ☛ Set aside

- In the same blender, pulse your oatmeal until the same consistency
- In a bowl, combine ground oatmeal, cocoa butter, honey, and ground almonds
- Rub into your clean feet, step into cotton socks, and leave on overnight
- The next morning, remove the socks and rinse feet in cool water
- Pat dry
- We recommend you not remove the socks until you're standing in the tub

Almonds and oatmeal act as exfoliators, gentle on the skin, yet powerful to remove the dead skin. Oatmeal is hypoallergenic at the same time. Cocoa butter moisturizes and nourishes the skin, while honey adds an antibacterial touch to the whole mix. Great recipe!

COFFEE FOOT SCRUB

Ingredients

4 tablespoons of ground coffee (fresh is the best)
3 tablespoons of corn meal (or ground oatmeal)
3 tablespoons of sea salt or Epsom salt
3 tablespoons of Olive or Almond oil
2 drops of lavender oil (or peppermint if you don't need relaxing, but simply want some energy boost

Preparation
- ☞ Mix all the ingredients well
- ☞ Scrub your feet in circular motion
- ☞ Rinse off with warm water and pat dry

Foot soak recipes are a great way to pamper yourself after a hectic day. Pamper your feet and relax your mind.

New Organic Recipes To Treat Your Feet

Skin Care is an all over body process because your skin is the largest and most protective organ you have.

Your feet are especially vulnerable because they take constant abuse from friction and elements but they do not produce sebum, which is your bodys natural oil. These organic skin care recipes for feet are fabulous when used in conjunction with a good foot care schedule. With all of our recipes, we urge you to buy organic ingredients because your skin absorbs pesticides and commercial chemicals from non organic products.

HONEY CLEANSER

This mild organic cleanser is terrific for feet because of its natural moisturizing and antibacterial qualities. Wet your foot and apply 1 tablespoon organic clover honey to a warm, wet washcloth rub entire foot thoroughly, being sure to get between all toes and around toenails. Rinse thoroughly with warm water.

FOOT SOAKS

Foot soaks are an excellent way to care for the skin as well as add to your total sense of well being. They soften dry skin and energize tired feet. After soaking, moisturize with a good organic moisturizer (see our article on organic moisturizer recipes if you would like to make your own).

ENERGIZING FOOT SOAK #1

Add 4 cups warmed organic whole milk, 2 tablespoons Epsom Salt, 2 tablespoons organic almond oil and 3 drops organic peppermint essential oil to a warm water foot bath. Soak feet for 15 minutes.

ENERGIZING FOOT SOAK #2

Add 2 drops of organic lemon essential oil, 2 drops or organic rosemary essential oil, and 4 tablespoons organic oat flour to a warm water foot bath. Soak for 15 to 20 minutes.

RELAXING FOOT SOAK #1

Add 4 cups warmed organic whole milk, 2 tablespoons Epsom Salt, and 6 drops organic lavender essential oil to a warm water foot bath. Soak for 15 minutes.

RELAXING FOOT SOAK #2

Add 1/4 Epsom Salt, 1 teaspoon baking soda, 2 drops each of these organic essential oils: lemon, sandalwood, coriander to warm water foot bath. Soak for 15 to 20 minutes.

DRY FOOT SOAK #1

Use warmed whole organic milk and 3 drops organic lavender essential oil. Soak your feet for 15 to 20 minutes and follow with exfoliating treatment. Rinse well. Massage with a liberally applied heavy organic cream moisturizer and cover with cotton socks for the night.

DRY FOOT SOAK #2

Add 3 cups organic pineapple juice and 1/2 cup organic coconut milk to a warm water foot bath. Soak for 10 to 15 minutes and follow with an exfoliating treatment. Rinse well. Massage with liberally applied heavy organic cream moisturizer and cover with cotton socks for the night.

PERSPIRATION/ODOR RESISTANT SOAK

Add 6 drops of organic common tea tree essential oil to a warm water foot

bath and soak for 15 to 20 minutes. Dry
thoroughly to discourage fungal growth.
Tea Tree essential oil has antibacterial,
antifungal, and astringent properties
which eliminate the various causes of foot
odor. Exfoliation

All of the following exfoliation mixtures will work much better
if used immediately after one of the above foot soaks.

CITRUS SCRUB

Mix 1 cup Epsom Salt, 3 teaspoons organic
olive oil and the juice of one small
lemon. Immediately massage soles of
feet (don't give the Epsom Salt time to
dissolve), giving extra attention to
any areas of thick skin. Rinse with warm
water.

SOUR CREAM SCRUB

Rub just soaked feet with 1 cup organic
cornmeal then apply a mixture of 1/4 cup
organic sour cream and 2 tablespoons
organic olive oil. Massage well, giving
extra attention to thick skin. Rinse with
warm water.

HONEY

Honey foot recipes are just a few of the honey skin care recipes. They could easily become a regular part of foot pedicure routine. Honey is a natural antiseptic that cleanses the skin deeply while keeping in check any possible inflammations and infections.

Your feet bear your weight day in and day out. Your feet can also feel stressed out and tired. When pampering your feet, you can opt for honey foot recipes, recipes for a natural pedicure which helps in elimination of the accumulated toxins and rejuvenation of feet.

This following uses honey in all stages. The honey that you use should be organic and produced locally for best effects. (Vegans can skip on the honey or opt for a little organic agave nectar.)

- Foot recipes - All-natural detox
- Black tea (fair trade brands): 2 bags
- Honey: 1 tea spoon
- Lemon: 1 tea spoon
- Hot/ warm water: 1 bucket

Mix all the ingredients in hot water. Let your feet soak in it for about ten minutes. Remove the dead skin by using a pumice stone. Then, make a foot scrub as given below.

- Honey foot scrub
- Hawaiian or any sea salt: 1 cup
- Honey: 1 teaspoon
- Coconut or any oil: 3 table spoons

Mix all the ingredients and then rub them on your feet. Make sure you cover the achy spots too. You can even massage this preparation on your hands too. Use warm water to rinse it off.

MOISTURIZING SALVE

Honey: a couple of table spoons (you can find some good deals in the farmers market)

Coconut oil: a couple of tea spoons (alternatively you can try sweet almond oil)

Mix these ingredients in a bowl. When you scrub and detox, you can put the bowl in a bigger vat of warm water to heat the mix. Rub it generously on your feet and keep it on for the next 15 minutes. You can use old socks or saran wrap to wrap your feet up for better results. After fifteen minutes, use warm water and organic soap to rinse off.

Chapter 9

Conclusion

Please remember, the publication of this information does not constitute the practice of medicine, and this information does not replace the advice of your physician or other health care provider. Before undertaking any course of treatment, the reader should seek the advice of his or her physician or other health care provider.

Like the rest of your body, your feet need great care to stay healthy and fit. Following a basic cleansing routine is essential to preserve the health of your feet. By keeping your feet clean and hygienic, you are actually protecting them from unwanted and distressing foot diseases.

Nature has provided humankind with a bounty of healthy, enriching, and nourishing oils and herbs to banish infection and keep the skin glowing. Natural remedies are both effective and safe for prolonged use. Since these simple remedies are very therapeutic and inexpensive, they save you a fortune! These home remedies have proved their worth over the ages. The dawn of modern medicine has not dimmed their reputation as the most cost-effective, soothing, safe, and healing treatments for foot conditions.

The natural foot care remedies discussed in this book are from an array of nature-based remedies collected from diverse websites. Most have been tested by time and proven to be highly beneficial for treating specific conditions.

These natural treatments are easy to follow and require minimal effort on your part to implement them. Since most of the ingredients are found right in your kitchen cupboard and backyard garden, your task is easy. A few highly active natural ingredients like ginger, garlic, Epsom salts, kosher salt, turmeric, coconut oil, cornstarch powder, berries, and herbs are adequate to treat many foot problems. You can explore the goldmine of other equally marvelous natural ingredients that are just as effective when it comes to treating common foot problems of all kinds.

As the popular saying goes, "An ounce of prevention is better than a pound of cure." The earlier you start caring for your feet, the lower your risk is of having to deal with serious foot problems.

Why couldn't the hikers cross the footbridge?
It had fallen arches!

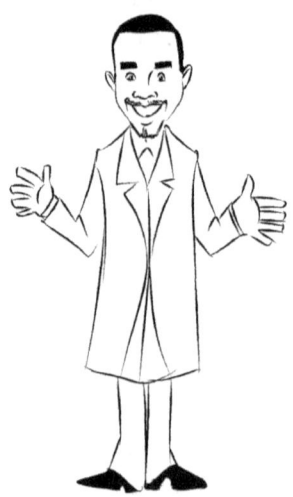

Glossary

Abrasive: Having a property of rubbing or grinding.

Acrylic: A synthetic fiber made from acrylate polymer.

Acupressure: Traditional Chinese massage technique that involves using the natural energy of your body to help heal pain.

Aloe Vera: A plant with thick fleshy leaves used widely in traditional medicine for its cooling and hydrating properties.

Analgesic: Having the property of relieving pain.

Anthocyanin: A blue, violet, or red plant pigment.

Antioxidants: Substances capable of preventing or reversing cell damage due to oxidation.

Astringent: A substance that tightens up body tissues, especially the skin.

Borage seed oil: Oil obtained from Borago officinalis, having anti-inflammatory properties.

Boswellia: A tree yielding a fragrant oil which has anti-inflammatory properties.

Bunion pads: Soft gel or fleece pads used to support and protect bunions.

Cayenne: A pungent spicy herb belonging to the pepper family.

Charcot foot: Charcot foot is a condition causing weakening of the bones in the foot that can occur in people who have significant nerve damage (neuropathy).

Chilblains: Small, itchy, painful lumps that develop on the skin as an abnormal response to cold.

Cramp: A sharp, painful muscle contraction.

Decant: To pour off clear liquid solution from a mixture leaving the solid part undisturbed.

Dystrophic: Toenails that are brittle, discolored, and that grow excessively thick due to injury or infestation of several organisms.

Eczema: An allergic skin condition in which the skin breaks open with a sticky clear discharge.

Emery board: An abrasive tool usually used for reducing fingernails or toenails.

Epsom salt: An inorganic salt containing magnesium, sulfur and oxygen that can be used as a beauty product. It can also be used to soothe sore muscles when dissolved in water

Essential oils: Oils extracted from herbs and seeds that possess various medicinal properties.

Eucalyptus oil: The pungent oil obtained from the eucalyptus tree, with a warming and mucus-clearing action.

Exfoliation: The removal of superficial dead layers of the skin.

Fenugreek: Mediterranean and Asiatic herb with aromatic seeds, used around the world as a culinary spice. It is soothing to the stomach. Other external formulations have been used for wounds and skin irritations.

Fibroma: An overgrowth of fibrous tissue into a mass.

Flip-flops: A kind of open-toed footwear held to the foot by thongs.

Floaters: A kind of casual open footwear with straps over the foot and ankle.

Gel: A thick, jelly-like substance.

Gel cap, gel pad: A gel covering for the toes to prevent rubbing and friction against footwear.

Heating pad: A pad that produces heat by electricity or chemical reaction, and is used to warm parts of the body.

Heel Spur: When the heel is exposed to constant stress, calcium deposits build up forming small bone spurs located on the bottom of the heel bone.

Hypertension: A condition where the blood pumps through the blood vessels at too high a pressure and can damage them as well as other organs.

Hypothyroidism: A condition in which the body becomes swollen and sluggish due to lack of the essential secretion from the thyroid gland in the front of the neck.

Inflammation: Swelling, redness, and pain in a part of the body associated with a response to a chemical or other toxic stimulus.

Interphalangeal: Located between the bones that make up one finger or toe.

Kosher salt: A coarse-grained salt without additives.

Lecithin: A fatty substance rich in choline and phosphorus. An excellent emulsifier and said to have health benefits.

Ligament: The tough fibrous tissue that holds the bones in a joint together.

Metatarsal: The bones that attach the fingers or toes to the wrist or ankle.

Metatarsalgia: Localized pain in the ball of the foot.

Moisturizing, moisturizer: Having the property of adding and locking in moisture in the skin.

Multiple sclerosis: A nerve condition causing weakness and paralysis of the body.

Natural fabric: Fabric woven from natural materials like cotton, cotton silk, or flax.

Nerve tonic: A medicine that stimulates the nerves in a healthy way.

Neuropathy: Disease process of the nerves, often causing weakness, numbness and pain, usually located in the hands and feet.

Nylon: A synthetic fiber.

Omega 3 fatty acids: Vital for normal metabolism. Some of the potential health benefits for normal body functions include controlling blood clotting and building cell membranes in the brain. Our bodies cannot make omega-3 fats, so we must get them through food.

Orthotic: A device meant to support and strengthen weak joints or bones.

Over-pronation: The movement in which the ankle rolls inwards too far.

Pancreas: An organ near the small intestine that produces digestive enzymes and hormones like insulin.

Pedicure: The process of improving the appearance of the feet and toenails.

Peripheral arterial disease: A disease process in which arteries to the limbs are blocked, resulting in poor limb circulation.

Plantar fibromas: An overgrowth of fibrous tissue into a mass found on the bottom of the foot.

Podiatrist, podiatry: A branch of medicine dealing with ailments of the foot and ankle.

Potassium: A soft mineral involved in many cell functions.

Pumice: A light volcanic stone widely used for scrubbing off dead skin.

Pumps: High-heeled shoes.

Purines: Natural substances found in all of the body's cells, and in virtually all foods. Uric acid is the chemical formed when purines have been broken down.

Raynaud's phenomenon: Excessively reduced blood flow in response to cold or emotional stress, causing discoloration and coldness of the fingers, and toes.

Rayon: An artificial, non-absorbent fiber.

Salon: An establishment run by a hairdresser, clothier, or beautician.

Sandals: An open type of outdoor footwear with straps or thongs.

Sea salt: Salt obtained from evaporation of seawater.

Silicone: A polymer that can withstand temperature changes and chemical attack or reaction.

Slippers: A comfortable slip-on shoe.

Sodium: A soft mineral involved in many cell processes, notably the transmission of nerve impulses.

Spa: A tub for relaxation. Also, a resort with therapeutic services such as massages, saunas and pedicures.

Spore: A highly resistant reproductive body produced by bacteria and fungi.

Sprouted legumes: Pulses (legumes, pea family) that have been allowed to sprout for a few days in clean, controlled conditions to become more nutritious.

Sunscreen: Chemicals that can prevent the action of solar radiation on the skin.

Tendon: The part of the muscle that attaches to bone.

Tendonitis: Inflammation of the tendon.

Toe crest: A device to hold deformed toes down and prevent their rubbing against footwear.

Toe Separators: Cushions or material placed between the toes, intended to reduce friction and irritation, used for medical conditions and spas.

Toe spreader: A device to hold toes apart and prevent them from overlapping.

Tumor: An abnormal growth of cells that forms a mass.

Turmeric: A yellow spice with anti-inflammatory properties.

Unsaturated fatty acid: A chemical that forms the building blocks of fats that are low in hydrogen content.

Uric acid: A chemical formed when purines have been broken down. The accumulation of uric acid crystals is called gouty arthritis, or simply "gout".

UV: Stands for ultra violet – that part of the light spectrum that is beyond human vision.

Varicose veins: A condition in which veins become dilated and distorted due to the failure of the valve system inside them.

Yoga: An Eastern system of mind and body control involving meditation and physical exercises.

CREDITS

hope you enjoyed my book. Even though I would love to take the credit for all this incredible and insightful natural foot care information, I must acknowledge all the websites where I was able to extract good healthy foot tips and facts.

http://clubfootclub.org/ (Riddles)
http://www.emedicinehealth.com
http://www.medicinenet.com
http://www.earthclinic.com
http://www.drweil.com
http://frugallysustainable.com
http://www.life-saving-naturalcures-and-naturalremedies.com
http://www.thriftyfun.com
http://www.alternativz.co
http://www.drweil.com
http://www.patient.co.uk
http://www.medicinenet.com
http://www.nhs.uk
http://www.webmd.com
http://www.yournextstep.net
http://arthritis.about.com
http://www.wvu.edu
http://www.foot.com
http://www.footsolutions.com
http://www.thepedicureroom.com
http://books.google.co.in
http://www.50plus-fitness-walking.com

http://www.ehow.com
http://www.top10homeremedies.com
http://www.footankle.com
http://www.readersdigest.ca
http://www.footvitals.com
http://diabetes.webmd.com
http://www.daveshealingnotes.com
http://www.realsimple.com
http://www.heel-that-pain.com
http://www.canadianliving.com
http://yourhealthybody.jillianmichaels.com
http://beta.active.com
http://www.everydayhealth.com
http://health.howstuffworks.com
http://www.naturesnaturalhealing.com
http://www.naturalnews.com
http://www.vidavibrante.com
http://health.howstuffworks.com/wellness/natural-medicine
http://www.wikipedia.com
http://www.boldsky.com
http://www.skin-care-recipes-and-remedies.com
http://www.Spaindex.com

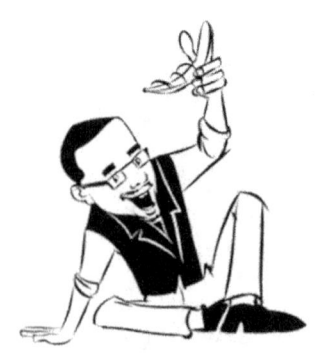

About the Author

Dr. Maasi J Smith was born in 1969 and is a native of New Jersey. He has lived in the Philadelphia area for the last 20 years.

Dr. Smith received his Doctor of Podiatric Medicine degree from Temple University's School of Podiatric Medicine in Philadelphia, Pennsylvania, 1999. He is also a graduate of Hampton University, 1992. Currently, he is a Podiatric Surgeon, who serves the community at Urban Health Initiatives of South Philadelphia. Dr. Smith is also a medical contributor to local and national television and radio.

Feet Naturally is the first in a series of books that will discuss nature's benefits for your feet.

He is the father of two beautiful daughters, Noelle and Nyla, who live in New Jersey.